Rationing in the NHS

Principles and pragmatism

Rationing in the NHS

Principles and pragmatism

Bill New
Senior Research Officer, King's Fund Policy Institute

Julian Le Grand
*Richard Titmuss Professor of Health Policy,
London School of Economics, and Professorial Fellow,
King's Fund Policy Institute*

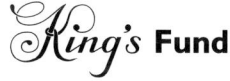

Published by
King's Fund Publishing
11–13 Cavendish Square
London W1M 0AN

© King's Fund 1996

First published 1996

All rights reserved. No part of this publication may be reproduced, stored in a retrieval system or transmitted, in any form or by any means, electronic or mechanical, photocopying, recording and/or otherwise without the prior written permission of the publishers. This book may not be lent, resold, hired out or otherwise disposed of by way of trade in any form, binding or cover other than that in which it is published, without the prior consent of the publishers.

ISBN 1 85717 113 6

A CIP catalogue record for this book is available from the British Library

Distributed by Bournemouth English Book Centre (BEBC)
PO Box 1496
Poole
Dorset
BH12 3YD
Tel: 0800 262260
Fax: 0800 262266

Printed and bound in Great Britain by Peter Powell Origination & Print

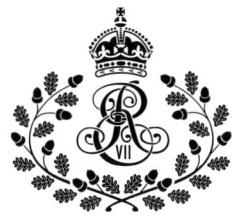

Contents

Acknowledgements vii

1 Introduction 1
2 Rationing in practice 5
3 Can rationing be more rational? 23
4 Principles of rationing: what's on the menu? 31
5 Principles of rationing: choosing between people 55
6 Conclusion 69

References 73

Acknowledgements

We would like to thank many of our colleagues at the King's Fund Policy Institute who read and made valuable comments on earlier drafts of this book, especially: Jennifer Dixon, Anthony Harrison, Ken Judge, Nicholas Mays and Sue Shouls. We would also like to thank David Mechanic and Rudolf Klein for helpful discussions on many of the topics.

Chapter 1

Introduction

A number of recent high-profile cases have brought the issue of rationing health care to public attention. Perhaps the most famous is that of Child B, who was denied treatment for leukaemia by her health authority allegedly on the grounds of cost. But there were several previous cases that attracted similar publicity, summarised in Box 1. Partly as a result of such cases, there is now a growing awareness in a variety of quarters that the rationing of health care is unavoidable. With the advance of medical technology, rising incomes and a general growth in health awareness, the demand for health care is growing faster than the resources allocated to it. And if more people want more care than can be met from available resources, then a process has to take place that decides who should get what. That is the rationing process, and it is one that, in the circumstances described, is widely seen to be inevitable.

> **Box 1: Rationing and the media**
>
> In April 1994, the BBC *Today* programme uncovered a 73-year-old man who had been denied physiotherapy by a hospital because he was over 65 – a policy that had been outlined in a letter to GPs in the area. The director of the physiotherapy unit in the hospital was quoted as saying that 'there has to be a cut-off point' and that people below 65 would be more likely to be at work and would need to get better more quickly. In 1993, Harry Elphick, a heavy smoker, was denied treatment for a heart condition on the grounds of his inability to quit smoking; he was the focus of a television programme, *The Heart of the Matter*. He died shortly afterwards. More recently, a letter in *The Lancet* in August 1995 claimed that elderly people were being denied palliative treatment for lung cancer on the grounds of their age (Hickish *et al.*, 1995). In the same month, Berkshire Health Authority leaked a plan to stop purchasing 12 treatment procedures, including treatment for varicose veins, removal of wisdom teeth, insertion of ear grommets and dilation and curettage (D&C). All these stories attracted extensive national media coverage and comment.

However, until recently there was little sustained analysis of the possible principles that might underlie this process. A number of publications in the last two years in a variety of countries have begun to fill this gap (BMJ, 1993; National Advisory Committee, 1994; Frankel and West, 1993; Dunning, 1992; Harrison and Hunter, 1994; Health Care and Medical Priorities Commission, 1993; House of Commons Health Committee, 1995; Maxwell, 1995). However, the overall result is a confusing picture; this book is an attempt to organise some of the relevant arguments into what is hoped is a more coherent one.

There are two, rather different, kinds of question that have been commonly confused in rationing discussions. The first concerns *what* should be rationed; the second, *who* should receive priority, or how should rationing be conducted between people.

The *what* question relates to the package or range of treatments or services that are to be provided free in a publicly funded system such as the UK National Health Service (NHS). What should be included in this package and what should be excluded? Should, for example, *in vitro* fertilisation, tattoo removal, dentistry and community care be provided free? Should they be left for people to purchase out of their own resources from private providers of various kinds? Or should there be some kind of half-way house where the service is provided free for some but not for others (such as a means-tested service giving free provision for the poor, but charged-for provision to the better-off)? Put another way, the issue here is what should be rationed through the price system, as with most other goods and services in the economy, and what through non-price rationing mechanisms.

The *who* question concerns rationing between individuals. If we conclude that some treatment or services will be provided free or largely so, then it is likely that, as with any good provided free, more of the services concerned will be demanded than is available. In that case, who should receive the service, and who should be denied it? Alternatively put, if providing a service or treatment free means that there is a queue for that treatment or service, who should go to the head of the queue and who to the back?

Within both the *what* and the *who* questions, there are further issues. First, in each case, we could ask who should make the relevant decisions. Thus in the *what* case, should it be the central government, local purchasers, professionals, or the public, who decides what is to be provided free under the NHS and what is not? In the *who* case, should it be clinicians, managers, civil servants, philosophers, economists, tax-payers, or patients themselves who decide on priorities?

As will become apparent, the question as to who decides is not easily separated from the other issues involved in the rationing debate. However, we shall begin by concentrating on a second set of issues, again applicable to both the *what* and *who* types of question. These concern the *criteria* for making decisions. Regardless of who is making the decisions in each case, what should be the criteria for making them? On what principles should decision-makers base their rationing decisions? To what extent should those principles be tempered with pragmatism?

Some people might argue that any such enterprise is foolish. The decisions concerned will be based in large part on the values of the decision-maker; and values, by definition, cannot be the subject of rational discussion. Hence the only meaningful discussion is over who will make the decisions; not over how the decisions should be made. However, this is not a view we share. While it may be true that people have ultimate values that are not amenable to logical argument, there is still plenty of room for rational analysis. In particular, there is considerable confusion over precisely what principles should underlie what kinds of decisions; there is also a lack of clarity in defining the principles themselves. Part of the aim of this analysis is to rectify these problems.

Chapter 2 offers a brief discussion of rationing in practice. Chapter 3 discusses whether rational, in the sense of explicit, systematic and democratic, rationing is possible at all; and if it is possible, whether it is desirable. Chapter 4 addresses the *what* question, and discusses some of the principles that might be useful in deciding what should be 'on the menu' under the NHS and what should not. Chapter 5 discusses the *who* question, again evaluating alternative principles. Chapter 6 provides a summary of the principal points.

Chapter 2

Rationing in practice

Rationing may be inevitable, but it can be achieved in a number of different ways. In this chapter, we review the traditional NHS method for allocating resources, the pressures which have promoted change and some examples of 'rational' rationing.

Origins

The need for rationing was not always recognised by the architects of the NHS. Indeed, in 1948 it was thought that as the NHS developed, the need for spending on health care would diminish as existing ill health was 'mopped up'. At the time, ill health was in large measure the result of easily curable diseases such as tuberculosis and poliomyelitis. But the eradication of such killer diseases merely revealed a deeper well of ill health in other forms. As premature deaths were reduced, an ageing population increasingly suffered from chronic, often incurable, conditions such as cancer and cardiovascular conditions (Klein, 1993b). Technological advance could ameliorate or 'repair' such conditions, but it did not reduce the demand on resources; on the contrary, the outcome of many of these interventions left a continuing need for care, and even when particular conditions were truly cured, others took their place – a process which shows no signs of abating (Callahan, 1994).

It very quickly became obvious to the NHS's political masters that, because of these pressures, the NHS would be permanently faced with demands that would exceed the resources allocated to meet them. The immediate response of governments to this dilemma in the first years of the NHS included imposing charges and capping the budget (Klein, 1995). Charges were levied for prescriptions, dental and optical services, both as a means of reducing demand and of increasing revenue. However, the financing system was otherwise open-ended, with the pressures on resources being met simply by supplementary estimates voted by Parliament. The system meant that expenditure could be increased within a financial year, so hospitals which ran out of money simply submitted claims for more. This was never likely to be politically sustainable, and in 1950 a ceiling was imposed on NHS hospital expenditure within any one year (family health service expenditure remained non-cash limited). Thus the fixed budget was born, and it has remained to this day the basis on which the NHS manages its financial affairs.

Cash-limiting required that hospital authorities had to work within their allocations: rationing had become a reality. But the administrative arrangements of the NHS were, from these early years in its development, characterised by a large degree of local autonomy. The centre would set the budget and issue broad guidance on the ends which were to be achieved, but the precise way in which resources were used for patient care was left to the periphery. Lack of information about what went on in individual hospitals, though, was criticised in early analyses of the NHS' financial workings as constituting a serious absence of accountability about how public money was spent:

> *The Ministry ... has no costing yardsticks at its disposal by which to judge the relative efficiency or extravagance of administration of various hospitals, and hence no alternative but either to accept the estimates wholesale as submitted without amendment, or to apply overall cuts to the total budgets in a more or less indiscriminate manner.* (Jones, 1950, quoted in Klein, 1995, p. 44)

Various initiatives from the centre did attempt to address these shortcomings, but without much success. Indeed, even after fixed budgets had been introduced, the allocation of these resources to hospital authorities remained largely based on inherited patterns of provision based, in turn, on the expenditure of the pre-NHS local health authorities (Klein, 1995). This tended to perpetuate a distribution which favoured the better-off areas. There were certainly no explicit criteria and, in the words of the Guillebaud report into the cost of the NHS, 'the main weakness of the present system for allocating revenue funds is the lack of a consistent long-term objective' (Cmd 9663, quoted in Klein, 1995, p. 47).

Although such criticisms were eventually addressed by explicit processes for geographical allocations, such as the work of the Resource Allocation Working Party (RAWP) and weighted capitation formulae, the way in which resources were used by hospitals and health authorities remained largely implicit. Again, historically determined patterns of service provision proved hard to change. Attempts by the centre to prioritise and reallocate resources – in favour of, for example, the so-called 'Cinderella' services for people with mental and physical disabilities, and elderly people – were often frustrated at the district health authority level where the medical profession enjoyed a significant influence (Ham, 1985).

If 'broad brush' reallocations proved difficult, the centre's influence over rationing at the hospital unit level – between acute specialties, for example – was negligible, and the workings of such rationing mechanisms that did exist mysterious and hidden from view. In a famous study by two US commentators, the British hospital was described as a:

> *quasi-feudal enterprise, ruled largely by a peerage of consultants ... [who] must parcel out the meagre rations allotted through the health district ... British consultants are responsible, directly or indirectly, for the disposal of almost all the hospital's resources. The typical British hospital administrator, unlike his US counterpart, has little power or authority in his institution.* (Aaron and Schwartz, 1984, p. 20)

Reforms to strengthen managers' position, particularly the Griffiths reforms, met with only limited success (S Harrison, 1988). Health care resources are still largely controlled by individual consultants managing waiting lists for those accepted for treatment. They decide which patients are admitted, when and for how long. There are no explicit criteria for this decision, which, along with decisions involving treatment, is the basis for the notion of clinical freedom.

In short, from the inception of the NHS in the 1940s, the rationing of scarce resources at all levels within the NHS has been largely controlled by the medical profession and has been implicit in nature, making no reference to agreed systems or criteria. While this still remains in large measure a reasonable summary of what happens in the 1990s, there is a growing perception that the pressures on health care systems have grown, not just in the UK (Turnberg, 1995; Healthcare 2000, 1995; House of Commons Health Committee, 1995) but internationally (Honigsbaum et al., 1995), and that systems of implicit rationing are due a reassessment.

Pressures

The implicit system of rationing hospital services described above survived without serious challenge for much of the first half century of the existence of the NHS. This is not to say that the NHS was never under serious financial pressure; on the contrary, it has always been so. Enoch Powell's observations (Powell, 1966, p.16) – based on his experience as a minister in the early 1960s – that what characterises the NHS is the 'deafening chorus of complaints' about funding levels, and the 'vested interest in denigrating' the service by those who work within it, have long been accepted as the conventional wisdom. Nevertheless, with the exception of the territorial allocation of national resources, there were no serious attempts fundamentally to alter the way the fixed budget should be rationed.

Implicit systems of rationing which claim universal and comprehensive care can continue to function as long as demand does not exceed supply by too great a margin. Whilst there are a number of recent commentators who question whether the NHS is indeed under increased pressure, or whether this is inevitable in the light of so much uncertain effectiveness (see, for example, Mullen, 1995), it is our judgement that the demands on, or 'expectations' of, the service will continue to grow as least as fast as the resources allocated to meet them. Such a judgement is backed by many in this country (see, for example, Harrison and Hunter, 1994) and echoes that of an eminent commentator in the USA, a country which is already spending far more than the UK on health care:

> *No matter how far we push the frontiers of medical progress we are always left with a ragged edge – with poor outcomes, with cases as bad as those we have succeeded in curing ... Whether it be intensive care for the premature newborn low birthweight baby, or bypass surgery for the very old, or AZD therapy for AIDS patients ... and when, eventually, those problems are solved there will be others to take their place.* (Callahan, 1994, p. 63)

This situation is arguably leading to a sea-change in attitudes. If the gap between demand and supply continues to widen, or at least persistently refuses to narrow, the NHS will be able to do less of what is expected of it, and may suffer a Habermas-type 'legitimation crisis'.[1] Such an outcome becomes more likely in the context of a better educated, better informed and less acquiescent citizenry. 'Patients' have been replaced with 'consumers', increasingly assertive about what they expect from the NHS and anxious to know why they are not getting it. The realisation is growing that people are denied treatment not because one has to wait one's turn or because 'there is no more that can be done', but because of the finite nature of resources. Under these circumstances, it could be argued, systems of implicit rationing can no longer sustain the myth that the NHS can do all things for all people. From the perspective of those working within the NHS, there is pressure to 'come clean' and admit to rationing explicitly.

Another response to an increasing gap between supply and demand is to improve the efficiency of the supply-side. Policies of this kind originated most notably from health economists, and greatly influenced the thinking of Conservative governments of the 1980s. However, the suggestion that health care resources could be allocated in a more rational and systematic way date back as far as the 1960s (see, for example, Klarman, Francis and Rosenthal, 1968). During the 1970s the economic techniques used in these analyses were refined, and one in particular – the Quality-Adjusted Life Year (QALY) – provoked widespread discussion among academics during the 1980s (see Williams, 1985). The simple proposition was that health systems such as the NHS, with their hidden and unmonitored resource allocation systems, were not getting the most from their resources. The health economists' arguments were characterised by a shift in focus from health 'inputs' – doctors, beds and hospitals – to 'outputs'. The NHS' output was hypothesised to be 'health': the more health which could be produced from the limited resources, the better. What was needed was improved information and resource allocation systems: to 'ration rationally' (Donaldson, 1993).

The increasing disparity between demand and supply and the influence of health policy analysts were both gradual processes. Indeed, despite government-led policies such as the Resource Management Initiative, the

---

1. Jurgen Habermas is a Marxist theorist who placed the crisis in modern capitalism, not in the economic sphere, but in the inability of the state to successfully reconcile its roles as a tax raiser, on the one hand, and distributor of benefits on the other. If this distribution is not seen as fair or in line with expectations, then there will be a deficit in legitimation (see Dumleavy and O'Leary, 1987, pp.264–5).

introduction of general management and the reorganisation of health authority structure, there was little change in the way resources were allocated as a direct result of these pressures. The catalyst for more significant change came with the enactment of the NHS and Community Care Act 1990, reforms implemented in 1991 and specifically directed at improving the efficiency of the service.

Under these reforms, responsibility for purchasing and providing health care services was split. Although not directly designed to make rationing more explicit, the reforms specifically sought to outline more clearly the respective roles of health authorities and provider units, though they said nothing about what was to be provided. On the one hand, health authorities were to assess the health needs of their population and purchase care best to meet that need; providers, on the other, were to compete for the contracts from the authorities. On both sides of the divide, health care agencies were encouraged to look more closely at how they could get the most from their resources. The complex hierarchical structure described above, wherein rationing was diffuse and unfocused, had been radically altered with potentially profound implications for the manner in which resources would be rationed in the future.

New ways of rationing

Developing new forms of rationing was not a specific government objective of the 1991 reforms. However, such forms did develop, largely as *ad hoc* responses to the reforms, and here we give some illustrations. The examples set out below give the impression of incoherence; this is not surprising given the absence of an overall strategy. However, they each display one or more characteristics which might be associated with rational behaviour. Clearly, what follows is somewhat of a contrived definition of 'rational', but it usefully sums up the various strategies which aim to 'do rationing better'. More precisely, these involve acting in a more explicit, systematic and democratic manner:

- *explicit* – practices are undertaken openly, even though they may have been in existence for many years;
- *systematic* – formal methodologies are designed for allocating resources consistently, usually involving a stipulation of the criteria to be used;

- *democratic* – the public are involved in the decision-making process, either directly or indirectly.

The examples are organised into three groups, depending on where in the NHS' hierarchy they originate: Department of Health, purchasers or providers. They are intended to give a flavour of the reaction of various agencies and individuals to the pressures on resources.

Department of Health initiatives

As indicated above, the Government does not have a coherent policy for introducing 'rational' rationing; however, this does not mean that they are averse to implementing initiatives which echo the general pattern. The two described here are included as they are unusually prescriptive, rather than being merely exhortatory.

Specification of maximum waiting times

Perhaps the most visible initiative has been the policy of reducing the numbers waiting for long periods for in-patient treatment. Prior to the 1991 reforms, the Government sought to address this problem with a centrally controlled fund, targeted at the 100 longest waiting lists in the country. After the reforms, the *Patient's Charter* introduced a new 'right' not to wait longer than two years from the time of first being placed on a waiting list for in-patient treatment. Both these policies explicitly emphasised that 'time waiting' was an important criterion for discriminating between those waiting, and, moreover, that once you had waited a very long period of time your claim on resources was substantially strengthened.

It has been argued that waiting lists 'blur' the true disparity between supply and demand in the NHS (Frankel and West, 1993). Better management and validation, administrative schemes such a booking system, practice guidelines and purchasing strategies could all substantially reduce the number waiting who can clearly benefit from, who genuinely want, and who are reasonably entitled to, treatment.

Nevertheless, whatever the real nature of the numbers waiting for treatment, it is highly significant that 'time waiting' should be accorded such a high priority. It is not self-evidently reasonable: encouraging health authorities to allocate resources to long waiters, who are not seriously ill, may divert resources from those more seriously ill. The President of the Royal College of Physicians was reported during the course of 1993 as saying that this was, indeed, happening and that urgent cases were on occasion delayed admission. Such issues point to the dangers of fixed systems perverting sensible decision-making in individual cases.

Excluding 'medicines' from NHS prescription

Much less widely publicised than waiting-list policies is the continuing effort by the government to restrict what GPs are free to prescribe on the NHS. For some time, the government has been adding to a 'limited list' of medicines excluded from NHS provision. Examples from the list are provided in Table 1.

Table 1

Medicines	*Pesticides and Toiletries*
Beecham Cough Capsules	Acarosan Foam
Flurex Bedtime Cold Remedy	Colgate Dental Cream
Unichem Cold Relief Capsules	Efamolia Night Cream
	Mitchell's Wool Fat Soap
Foods	SR Toothpaste
Gale's Honey	
Lambert's Evening Primrose Oil	
Rite-diet Diabetic Cherry Cake	
Schar Gluten Free Sponge Cake	

Source: A. Harrison, 1992, p.34

This initiative is an example of explicit rationing by exclusion, although it is not at all clear what the rationale for exclusion is, nor whether systematic criteria have been used. In some cases cost-effectiveness seems to have been the motive, as with the brand-name cold remedies, for example. In other cases, though, it appears that some intuitive judgement has been made. In a government minister's own words:

> The NHS should not be paying for items which have no therapeutic or clinical value. Items such as mineral water, cakes, lip salves and face powder cannot be classified as medicines. (Department of Health, 1993a)

But how can we clearly delineate between clinical and other values? The list itself fails to distinguish between criteria such as 'not being a medicine', not effective as a medicine, and cheap and simple remedies which could safely be left to personal responsibility. It is not, therefore, particularly rational or systematic. Nevertheless, the policy is highly explicit and provides an example of how national policy already exists for defining the boundary of the NHS.

Purchaser initiatives

The purchaser-provider split had, from a rationing perspective, the most profound implications for purchasing health authorities and GP fundholders. Freed from managerial responsibilities, health authorities were now faced with the task of making the best use of available resources to meet the health needs of their population. An opportunity was created to bring systematic analysis into play and move away from a process which largely reinforced the status quo.

Advisory committee on the ethics of purchasing strategies

As a response to the accusation that too much ethical analysis of purchasing dilemmas remains in academic circles, rather than positively contributing to the decision-making process, West Glamorgan Health Authority set up what they call a Local Ethics Committee (Purchaser Advice). Unlike more general ethics committees,

> *the LEC(PA) will concern itself with ethical issues arising out of resource allocation and other health care policy decisions; it will not be available for the immediate resolution of particular problems, either for the authority or its employees.* (Jarvis, 1994, p.17)

The Committee's members are drawn from a range of backgrounds, including professional philosophy, public health, dentistry, law, health service management and general practice; two members are from community health councils. All aspects of the health authority's spending plans will be submitted to the Committee for discussion and ethical review, although it will exercise no veto powers, the final responsibility for decisions remaining with the health authority itself.

The strategy adopted by the health authority reflects a belief that complex moral issues, as well as technical ones, can be subjected to systematic analysis, thereby improving the way such decisions are made. The approach also makes it explicit that rationing is taking place, and involves representatives of the local community. Precisely how systematic the discussions prove to be is another question – it is a large committee by modern standards – and its advisory status may simply allow the health authority to use it as evidence that it is taking its work seriously without actually absorbing its advice.

Use of cost-effectiveness evidence[2]

The use of cost-effectiveness evidence in decisions relating to the allocation of health care resources has already spawned a vast literature, and little can be usefully added in a short discussion such as this. However, it is worth dwelling briefly on the QALY and its use in systematic decision-making in the context of other initiatives described here. QALYs were referred to earlier in the context of professional analysts' influence on the development of rational rationing techniques. The rationale behind QALYs is that, subject to accurate evidence on the relative costs and benefits of various health care interventions, those interventions can be ranked in order of their cost-per-QALY. Interventions further up the list should, other things being equal, have higher priority.

In practice, however, QALYs had not demonstrated, pre-reform, that they had a significant impact on the decision-making process. To establish whether matters had changed in the post-reform era, the King's Fund Institute conducted a survey of the (then) 187 English district health authorities during the summer of 1992 (Robinson and New, 1992). Replies were received from 127, constituting a response rate of 68 per cent.

Twenty-one per cent of authorities replied that they had already used QALY evidence to assist decision-making, and a further 17 per cent unequivocally planned to do so. For a significant minority, therefore, QALYs have now become part of the rationing process. This finding

---

2. 'Cost-effective' is used here as a summary term to include notions of cost-utility and cost-benefit – particularly the ability to compare the effects of interventions on different states of ill-health. Although there are important differences between these measures, these distinctions do not affect the arguments in this book.

contrasts with that of Klein and Redmayne's (1992) study of purchasing plans, wherein there were no reported uses of QALY evidence. This is confusing, but may reflect a nervousness of individual authorities 'owning up' to using such a controversial technique so early in its development. The King's Fund survey preserved the anonymity of the respondents.

QALYs are clearly an attempt to be rather more systematic in how resources are allocated: not, as yet, by excluding non-cost-effective procedures but by influencing the priority given to interventions which display different degrees of cost-effectiveness. Their contribution to explicitness leaves much to be desired, however, with much of their use occurring behind closed doors and outside the view, or influence, of the general public. It is certainly not clear whether QALYs, or other health maximisation techniques, conform to what the public expect or desire from the NHS.

Fundholding practice advisory committee

GP fundholders have provoked a large measure of controversy as the 'wild card' in the purchasing pack, particularly as regards their potential for creating a two-tier service (Whitehead, 1994) and in the problems they create in retaining an integrated and coherent service. However, they also face a degree of criticism over their lack of accountability for how they use their funds (New, 1993). Little attention has been focused on the need to monitor the spending decisions of these agencies, given the control individual GPs have over large, and growing, proportions of the NHS hospital and community health services budget (Audit Commission, 1995).

Some fundholding practices have started to address these concerns on their own initiative. One practice in Suffolk has set up a public consultation group to help manage the fund and set treatment priorities (Feger, 1993). The six partners of the 10,000-patient practice asked 12 villagers to join the group, which then met the GPs to discuss clinical protocols and patients' views on waiting times for 180 procedures.

While such an initiative is an admirable attempt to address issues of explicitness and accountability, it also highlights the difficulty of implementing mechanisms which do not simultaneously 'skew' preferences toward vocal, articulate and influential members of the community. It was reported in this case, for example, that members of the committee included local authority councillors and an economist – not necessarily representative of 'ordinary' people. This problem will be returned to below.

Excluding 'minor' surgical procedures from NHS provision

During 1991, not long after the reforms were implemented, North East Thames Regional Health Authority was reported to have issued guidance that certain surgical procedures were no longer to be treated on the NHS, unless there was 'over-riding' need: the removal of non-malignant lumps and bumps, extraction of symptomless wisdom teeth, varicose vein operations, *in vitro* fertilisation and tattoo removal (Dean, 1991). Similarly, in comprehensive surveys of purchasing plans in 1992, 1993 and 1994/5, researchers at the University of Bath (Klein and Redmayne, 1992; Redmayne, Klein and Day, 1993; Redmayne, 1995) found that a small number of purchasers – no more than 12 in any one year – had removed certain minor procedures from NHS provision. The procedures concerned were similar to those excluded by North East Thames. And during 1995, Berkshire health commission circulated a document which was interpreted as suggesting that 12 procedures should be removed from NHS provision in order to address a funding shortfall (Crail, 1995).

Exclusions are, of course, highly explicit: the fact that procedures are no longer available on the NHS cannot be hidden from those seeking the service – although it has long been suspected that some waiting lists have been of a 'never never' variety, with consultants having little intention of ever providing treatment. Nevertheless, the *rationale* for excluding the services mentioned above was not made explicit, and indeed there is no indication that they were chosen with reference to any systematic set of criteria.

These exclusions did promote a degree of public controversy, out of proportion, perhaps, to the quantity of NHS expenditure which they represented. The procedures were all conducted on a small scale and were not, by and large, very expensive by NHS standards. However, the reason for public disquiet was a perceived weakening of the NHS' commitment to a comprehensive service. Perhaps in response to this controversy purchasing authorities appear to have become less willing to indulge in this form of rationing: the Bath research found that significantly fewer authorities had excluded procedures in the second year of their research than in the first, although the number rose again slightly in the third year. This finding surprised the researchers who had expected the 'exclusion policy' to continue and spread.

Furthermore, the North East Thames and Berkshire initiatives were both subject to official 'clarification' after the public uproar by those responsible for the relevant documents. Representatives from both authorities emphasised that they were not, in fact, proposing to withdraw services entirely and that where there was considered to be 'clinical need' they would still be provided. Indeed, in the Berkshire case, subsequent statements by those involved seemed to suggest that the strategy was merely an attempt to limit 'ineffective' treatments, and not to remove services because they were insignificant or could no longer be afforded (Crail, 1995).

These events contain a significance beyond the rather small quantity of NHS resources involved. It could be argued that purchasers were rather naive in circulating documents suggesting restricting the availability of certain treatments, even if the target was in fact only those that are ineffective. But there can be no doubt now that any strategy which could be interpreted as limiting the comprehensive nature of the NHS, if made explicit and poorly managed, will cause a public furore of considerable proportions.

Surveys of public opinion

After the publication of the government's *Local Voices* document in January 1992 (NHS Management Executive, 1992), many purchasing authorities pursued one or other of a number of consultation exercises to collect the views of their local populations. Some were more sophisticated and ambitious than others and aimed to evaluate how members of the community valued particular health states with a view to informing the prioritisation of services. One such survey, conducted among the residents of City and Hackney Health Authority, provoked much discussion during 1993, largely because of the mismatch between how members of the public and health professionals valued certain health services (Bowling, 1993). In particular, health professionals ranked services for mentally ill people, long-stay services and community-based services higher than the public, who, for their part, tended to favour life-saving interventions such as treatment for children with life-threatening illnesses.

The implication of these surveys will be analysed further below, although it is worth noting, and is perhaps unsurprising, that surveying the public did not provoke the same degree of controversy as those schemes which promote explicitness in how rationing is to be undertaken. Public opinion surveys are perceived as self-evidently 'good things', promoting democracy and responsiveness. However, those surveyed do not always approve of the goals of the strategy, that is, to assess how best to make use of limited funds. In response to a survey designed by the BMA and King's Fund, approximately half of the members of the public surveyed felt that funding should be unlimited (Heginbotham, 1993).

Provider initiatives

Although purchasers and central government might be expected to have most to gain from more rational rationing – providers, after all, need only to concern themselves with meeting contractual obligations – many hospitals and individual doctors have initiated policies which either made explicit existing practices, or developed more systematic methods for choosing patients for admission from waiting lists.

'Points' system

An initiative of a hospital in Salisbury operates in both an explicit and systematic manner, although the 'system', in its early stages, represents simply a formalisation of existing practice. Consultants were asked about the criteria they used when deciding when to admit patients; the results were transformed into a 'points' system under which patients were prioritised according to their score in five categories. The five categories were: speed of progress of the disease, pain or distress, disability or dependence on others, loss of occupation, and time waiting. Each could be scored from one to four points, depending on the condition and circumstances of the patient. The categories were not weighted or combined to produce an overall score, but simply used to provide a clear summary of each patient so that consultants could make better informed decisions, or target certain categories, such as those in severe pain or who were entirely dependent on others (Giles, 1993).

As currently organised, the Salisbury system is relatively unambitious – it simply formalises what already happens, with the significant difference that within a small number of specialties where the consultants have agreed to co-operate, decisions to admit patients are made openly on agreed criteria. However, such a scheme could become much more ambitious if the categories were weighted and the scores combined. This would further restrict discretion about who is to be admitted next. Furthermore, some patients could be excluded altogether. Alastair Lack, who runs the scheme, has been quoted as saying that, in due course:

> *if we've only got the funds to treat patients who score two or three or more, we're not going to put patients with minor conditions on the list.* (Giles, 1993)

Overall, the scheme raises questions about what the correct set of criteria are, how they should be combined, who allocates points, and under what circumstances clinicians should be allowed to 'trump' the scheme and exercise clinical freedom. But it also makes explicit what was implicit: if potential patients realise that they are being rated on various criteria – not all related to the seriousness of their condition – and therefore on their likelihood of admission, then such a scheme runs the risk of controversy of a similar magnitude to that caused by purchaser exclusions described above.

Excluding elderly people from certain forms of treatment

Rather than exclude patients on the basis of lack of severity in various categories, they can be excluded on the basis of a single characteristic such as age. Just such a policy has long been part of implicit rationing, and various studies have found age-related policies in stroke units, dialysis centres and transplant units (Dean, 1994). The example of the elderly man denied physiotherapy (described on page 1) led to a national outcry in response, with the Secretary of State forced to issue a press release indicating that 'the NHS provides services for everybody, on the basis of their clinical need and regardless of their ability to pay. There are no exceptions to this rule, whatever the age of the patient' (Department of Health, 1994).

Interestingly, the reason given for rationing by this criterion is rarely age *per se* – that the patient has already had a 'good innings' – but rather that age is a good proxy for other 'relevant' criteria, such as ability to benefit or being in work. The Secretary of State's statement seems to indicate that only clinical need/ability to benefit is an appropriate criterion: if being old means that you are less likely to benefit from treatment, then rationing is justified on this basis. Such a contention is always open to attack on empirical grounds; for instance, a study by Dudley and Burns (1990) found that some coronary treatment was more beneficial among elderly patients. What is clear, though, is that age alone is not considered a reasonable criterion – a conclusion echoed by a subsequent report which concluded that 'commissioning bodies should ensure that access for elderly patients to specialist (non-geriatric) facilities is as good as that for younger individuals, and that age is not used as an exclusion criterion in admission policies to specialist units' (Turnberg, 1994, p. 26).

However, some authors have specifically advocated that age should be adopted as a relevant criterion for rationing, based in part on the results of public opinion surveys (Lewis and Charny, 1989; see also Shaw, 1994). However, making such a policy explicit would clearly be extremely difficult from a political perspective, given the effect a single case had on the rationing debate.

Excluding individuals on the basis of their lifestyle

The question of whether or not one's choice of activities – or inactivities – should be taken into account when rationing decisions have to be made, caused a similar furore during 1993. The debate was sparked by the publication in the *BMJ* of an article which suggested that smokers should not be admitted for treatment of certain non-urgent heart conditions on the same basis as non-smokers because their chance of a successful outcome is severely reduced (Underwood *et al.*, 1993). The controversy gained further momentum from the death of Harry Elphick who had refused to stop smoking and was therefore not treated. The clinicians argued that an operation would have been ineffective; many others accused the doctors of exercising a judgement based on a particular lifestyle of which they disapproved. Again, the Government felt compelled to issue a press release, emphasising that clinical need was the only appropriate criterion (Department of Health, 1993b), while the British Medical Association emphasised that advice to give up smoking was indeed predicated on need and not lifestyle:

> ... it is of paramount importance that patients are not left with the impression that doctors ... are refusing to treat them. For some conditions giving up smoking can be the best immediate treatment. (British Medical Association, 1994)

As in many of the cases described in this chapter, the central issue is not so much that choices have to be made between those waiting for treatment – that has always been the case – but that choices are being made openly. This explicitness has exposed an absence of a clear, shared understanding of how choices should be made fairly and equitably.

Conclusion

The collective implication of the cases described in this chapter should not be exaggerated. The principal form of rationing in the NHS continues to be implicit and controlled by the medical profession. The public still have relatively little influence on how decisions are made. Purchasing health authorities and fundholders are by and large changing practice, if at all, cautiously. But there is every indication that they are set to continue to experiment, urged on by the exhortations of experts and by the hope that 'rational' progress will ease the financial pressures under which they work. The experience reviewed in this chapter is that such experiments will rarely provide uncontroversial solutions, and will often make a difficult situation worse. It is worth asking whether we can be more rational at all, and this question is the subject of the next chapter.

Chapter 3

Can rationing be more rational?

It should be clear from the examples in the previous chapter that moves toward explicit, systematic and democratic forms of rationing (what we term 'rational' rationing) are fraught with danger. Many of the initiatives were met with public outrage; those which were less well publicised have caused professional disagreement and controversy, albeit largely confined to the pages of specialist journals. But is this not rather surprising? After all, being explicit, systematic and democratic about any process would seem to be almost beyond reproach. Many of those involved in the examples described, particularly clinicians who opened up their practices, have been genuinely surprised at the reaction. Why is this?

Explicitness

Initiatives directed at opening up rationing practice are probably most at odds with traditional NHS methods. While it is now a commonplace to contend that rationing has always been present in the NHS, it is certainly not the case that the general public perceived that to be the case. The understanding was that all health care was available when it was needed; one individual was not to be discriminated in favour of another. Even the existence of waiting lists and the reality of the delays at the doctor's surgery were, it could be argued, perceived more as 'taking one's turn in the queue' than evidence that choices were being made between those making claims on public resources. After all, queuing is something we do when we wait for a bus, or when we wait at a supermarket checkout, and so would not suggest that there was any fundamental mismatch between supply and demand.

But, as we have seen, the situation is more serious than just a market sanctioned delay: it arises because the NHS cannot – and could not – do all that it claimed. The irony is that as those who worked within the NHS came to realise this, and attempted to be honest and open about it, the general public have seen it as a fundamental shift in public policy. Thus, attempts to exclude services, smokers or elderly people – no matter how 'rational' the thinking behind the attempts – were met with little short of outrage. The NHS, it seems, had successfully operated a benign deceit: patients had been willing to accept a doctor's (possibly disingenuous) assurance that 'nothing more can be done', but not the explicit denial that it is worth doing in the first place. As one commentator has put it:

> *The rush to embrace a greater degree of openness about the process of rationing health care ... is almost childlike in its innocence and naivety.*
> (Hunter, 1991, p. 20)

A national health care system, it might be argued, is less about producing health than public reassurance – what Bevan used to call 'tranquillity' (Dean, 1991). It reflects a contractarian rather than utilitarian notion of justice – that is, one which emphasises a complex, implicit agreement between the state and civic society, rather than one which focuses on explicit and supposedly measurable outputs. And, evidently, it is hard to design explicit processes which concord with an implicit contract – whatever it may be.

Systematic

Being more systematic about how health care is rationed has been most strongly supported by economists. Their arguments will not be rehearsed in detail here. But, in short, they viewed the NHS as charged with 'maximising health', and, indeed, believed that those working within it were working toward that goal; egalitarianism was the watchword for NHS activity only because implicit decision-making had obscured the NHS' goals (Culyer, 1988). In other words, individual decisions by those working within the NHS more closely reflected a maximising goal than an egalitarian one – in an emergency department, for example, when time was limited, the patient for whom most could be done would have priority. However, decisions such as these were not made according to systematic criteria.

Furthermore, cost-effectiveness techniques – including QALYs – should be 'complemented by consumer surveys, consensus conferences, meta-analyses', the purpose of which 'is to focus decision-makers' attention on the relevant information (cost-effectiveness) to inform rationing' (Sheldon and Maynard, 1993, p. 20). In fact,

> to ignore costs is <u>un</u>ethical because it means ignoring avoidable death and suffering. People who refuse to count the cost of their actions are not behaving <u>ethically</u>, they are behaving <u>fanatically</u>, and fanaticism has no place in the practice of medicine. (Williams, 1989, p.15, emphasis in original)

If there was a concern for equity, this concern should be explicitly built into prior systems based on health maximisation (Williams, in Bell and Mendus, 1988). The emphasis is squarely on outcomes – 'health gain' – with equity a matter of deciding on how that health should be distributed on explicit normative criteria.

These arguments in favour of designing formal systems for undertaking something as complex as rationing health care have been challenged by a number of commentators (Hunter, 1993; Harrison and Hunter, 1994; Klein, 1991 and 1993a). The criticisms are part of a wider literature challenging rationalist methods in the social sciences (Majone, 1989; Lindblom, 1979). The criticisms centre on the limitations of the factual information underlying the systems, their inability to accommodate all the complex and conflicting goals of public policy, and, in this context, their use as a substitute for political processes. Formal systems are also unable to provide guidance on individual cases.

The QALY has come in for the most criticism in this context. Certainly, information must be collected as well as possible so as to inform decision-making, and where decisions have to be made, they should be made with a clear view of the problem to be solved and the options available for solving them. But, if the contention that the NHS is a highly complex institution with many, often conflicting goals, is correct, then these systematic processes should have typically modest aims. If they attempt to 'solve' the grand problem of allocating resources within the NHS, they are likely to fall foul of one or other of the competing conceptions of what the NHS exists for. As one prominent proponent of economic evaluation puts it, health economists and their techniques should be 'on tap and not on top' (Robinson, 1993).

Even rather modest and apparently uncontroversial initiatives for being systematic in the practice of health care can suffer difficulties. In recent years there has been a growing interest in the use of clinical practice guidelines – systematic statements to assist clinicians in making decisions about appropriate health care in specific clinical circumstances. The guidelines form part of a wider movement to promote evidence-based medicine which, in the simplest terms, seeks to promote the use of interventions which work – which are clinically effective. While the development of guidelines has been broadly welcomed (Grimshaw and Hutchinson, 1995), there have been difficulties encountered with local acceptance. Part of the problem is that some clinicians may feel that guidelines restrict clinical freedom and are insufficiently flexible to accommodate individual circumstances (Mechanic, 1995). Certainly, if purchasing agencies were to use guidelines as part of the commissioning process to restrict the availability of certain treatments altogether, then this would weaken the ability of the individual clinician to decide on the effectiveness of a treatment on a case-by-case basis.

Whatever the future of clinical guidelines, the QALY, or other attempts to rationalise decisions about how best to use resources, these issues certainly serve to highlight the difficulties involved in implementing any systematic procedure in a highly complex, heterogeneous institution such as the NHS. They also remind us that those who promote such approaches – in this case, economists – may not be seen as having a legitimate role to play in the workings of an institution not generally associated with their academic discipline.

Democratic participation

Democratic participation might seem to be the least contentious of the moves toward rational systems of rationing. However, directly involving the public in the decision-making process carries significant dangers, although not of the kind that is likely to cause a public outcry – after all the 'public' are unlikely to oppose moves which seek their opinion. Nevertheless, the 'public' in this context are not simple to identify, let alone consult, and their wishes can prove hard to interpret.

The City and Hackney Health Authority and the GP fundholding committee experiences described above highlight the difficulties of gaining a representative sample of people to participate in resource allocation decisions. In City and Hackney, community services, those for mentally ill people and long-term care – for some of the most vulnerable members of the community – were ranked lower than expensive life-saving interventions. There must be a concern that in any such meeting the advice gained from the public will emanate from only one section of the population, usually the most affluent, vocal and articulate.

But even if perfectly representative samples of the public can be consulted, the legitimacy of their having a direct influence on resource allocation and rationing will still be deeply problematic. The outcome of such exercises will reflect majority opinion and, although it is hard to be sure what that opinion would be, it is likely that the interests of very old, infirm, mentally ill or disabled people will be neglected in favour of the concerns of the majority. High-technology rescue or repair medicine, for example, can more easily be conceived as immediately relevant to us all. Furthermore, it is simply naive to suppose that the lay public have the requisite knowledge to make many decisions which are of a complex, technical nature.

The traditional method for addressing such issues is representative democracy, whereby officials are appointed or elected to be responsible for taking and implementing decisions on behalf of the whole community. Encouraging direct decision-making by community groups would, it might be argued, constitute a fundamental break with this tradition, and would have the unfortunate consequence of allowing public officials to absolve themselves of the consequences of their actions, claiming that they simply 'did what the public wanted'.

Political decision-making – and that is what rationing decisions are – must be open to challenge, scrutiny and debate, and those who make the decisions must bear the responsibility for and deal with the consequences of those decisions. If not, poor decision-making can result. Why, for example, should members of the public make considered judgements when they do not face the prospect of being challenged on them, nor of answering for any unfavourable consequences? Accountability would, under these circumstances, be weakened. Political decisions will always be a compromise, arbitrating between different groups in society, made by people who represent the whole community and not just one set of interests. The general 'public' are not accountable in this sense. Thus, while the public must constitute one part of a system of representative democracy – that of scrutineers, consultants and ultimate arbiters of who should represent them – they should be involved to a greater degree with caution.

Incrementalism

The difficulties encountered in trying to implement initiatives aimed at promoting explicit, systematic and democratic rationing within the NHS are predictable, according to one theory of public sector decision-making. Known as 'incrementalism', the theory argues that for complex social problems, 'synoptic' analysis – analysis which attempts to be complete – is bound to fail since it is beyond the resources of any individual, research team or committee. As its chief proponent puts it:

> *The choice between synopsis and ... incrementalism ... is simply between ill-considered, often accidental incompleteness on one hand, and deliberate, designed incompleteness on the other.* (Lindblom, 1979, p. 519)

We should not even aspire to grand strategies or solutions. Furthermore, analysis and policy-making should consist of 'no more than small or incremental possible departures from the status quo' (ibid., p. 519). Policy-making can move fast and radically, but should do so in small manageable steps. Connected with incrementalism as policy analysis, is political decision-making as partisan mutual adjustment. This process involves the greatly decentralised and fragmented decision-making between many different participants, all bringing their own analysis and persuasive capabilities to bear on a multitude of problems, and coming to a decision by a process of bargaining and 'mutual adjustment'. This, it is argued, constitutes the best way for decisions to be made when the goals are highly complex, value-laden and contestable. Policy 'happens' rather than is made; rational analysis is not abandoned but squarely subordinated to a political process.

It must be said that QALYs, for example, are only proposed as aids to decision-making, as are moves to incorporate the public in decision-making. They are not often defended as grand solutions. Explicitness, too, has only been attempted in a small number of ways. Overall, indeed, 'priority setting ... continues for the most part to be implicit, as does the consequent rationing' (Redmayne, Klein and Day, 1993, p. 36). The insight of the incrementalist position, however, is to help understand why these schemes and initiatives cause so much consternation; why even hesitant, apparently modest attempts at changing how the NHS conducts the rationing of resources appear to throw those who work in the NHS, and those who see themselves as its guardians, into turmoil.

Conclusion

Although the incrementalist position offers insights into the difficulties involved in reforming an institution such as the NHS, it does not in itself offer solutions to the question of reconciling the expectations of those using it with its ability to satisfy them. There is no going back to the old NHS, and few would wish to return to a situation where rationing was conducted hidden from public view, largely governed by historical conditions and 'shroud waving', and undertaken by professionals uninformed of the costs and benefits associated with their decisions. Moreover, the public are becoming increasingly well informed about rationing issues as a fast-growing media industry deploys its considerable resources towards revealing and communicating stories of unmet need and denied treatment. Although such stories are not always presented in a balanced manner, they are rarely entirely manipulative: hard choices are indeed being made and will continue to be made regardless of the level of financing.

It therefore seems inevitable that there will be a continuing imperative to improve the way rationing is conducted. So what is to be done? At the very least, those tasked with rationing need better guidance. One strategy would be to outline principles – rather than codified systems or wholesale explicitness – which can be commonly agreed, and which can then be used to hold practitioners to account. Some principles – such as supporting only effective treatments – have already succeeded in achieving a large degree of consensus. Others are still the subject of significant controversy. Can any further progress be made? The next two chapters address themselves to the issues involved in trying to develop such principles, and suggest what some of those principles might be.

Chapter 4

Principles of rationing: what's on the menu?

As we have seen, the decisions by which health care resources are distributed between competing claims are becoming increasingly explicit. One category of decision-making, however, stands apart from the others. It focuses not on how to distribute resources between a range of competing options (treatment groups or individual patients), but on what constitutes the range itself. Whereas repeated statements of the NHS' mission refer to the universal provision of a comprehensive package of health care services, largely free at the point of use, precisely what constitutes that package is never spelt out.

Services are not always free at the point of use in the NHS. Some are charged at such a high proportion of their cost that universal provision has become little more than a minimal universal subsidy: dentistry is an example. In fact, conceptualising the issue in terms of 'free' or 'not free' is unhelpful, since there are a range of costs associated even with 'free' services with which users are faced, such as those associated with travel and treatment time. 'Universal' or 'non-universal' is more useful, since this distinction relates to the boundary between what the NHS does and what other agencies and the private sector do. Universal services are defined as those which are offered to everyone, regardless of income, at a subsidised price (generally zero) at the point of use. The question addressed in this chapter, therefore, is: What is, and what should be, the range of universally provided health services?

Of course, it is not the actual provision – in terms of state ownership of hospitals – which is of interest. The ill-fated Clinton proposals for a national health care system in the USA did not propose the socialisation of provision. But they did propose that everyone enrol in the scheme – a form of universal compulsion. In the UK, the arguments of this chapter could equally well apply if the private sector took over responsibility for the delivery of health care, as long as its finance remained under the public control of health authorities. The use of the term 'provision' should be taken to cover any of these mechanisms by which governments can ensure the availability of a service.

'Restricting the menu'

A strategy which attempts to ration by limiting the range of health care services available has been termed 'restricting the health care menu' (Klein, 1994). Occasionally, the term 'explicit rationing' is used to refer to these strategies (Klein and Redmayne, 1992), although, as is made clear in Chapter 5, how decisions are made between individuals can also be highly explicit. Nevertheless, defining the package of health care services, or those which are excluded, is a strategy worthy of analysis in its own right.

There are at least three identifiable approaches to 'restricting the menu': only provide those services which are proven to be effective; only provide those which are relatively cost-effective; or only provide those which are 'relevant' to a health care system.[1] The last strategy might seem unfamiliar, although the variants may not be: is the service concerned with 'health' benefits rather than other forms of benefit? Is it 'necessary'? Can it be left to the individual's responsibility? And so on. The report from the Dunning Committee in Holland cited the last two, along with effectiveness and cost-efficiency, as their guiding principles, but without managing to be specific about the services which might be excluded (Dunning, 1992; van de Ven, 1995). In New Zealand, the Core Services Committee, which advises the government on the fairest and most effective way of using public money for health care, attempted a similar strategy – although they did not find the task an easy one:

> ... in something of an anti-climax, the Committee recommended that 'core' be defined as being what was already being provided prior to the reforms .... [the Committee had] 'not found any treatment or area of service within the current range which can be completely excluded.'
> (Cooper, 1995, p. 805)

---

1. A fourth approach, sometimes included in these discussions, involves restricting services which people bring on themselves; however, such an approach sits more easily within the analysis of how to choose between people, and will be discussed in Chapter 5.

Clearly, defining what should be on the menu is not straightforward, though it will be argued in this chapter that one reason for this has been an inability properly to distinguish the three approaches mentioned above. But before analysing these approaches, it is worth reflecting a little on why these attempts were made in the first place. Why are 'boundary' issues important?

Issues surrounding the range of services provided by the NHS are important for two reasons. First, a desire for equity or fairness requires the provision of health services broadly in response to need. In a large public organisation such as the NHS, decisions relating to the level of provision of particular services are left to local decision-makers: health authorities or individual clinicians. Service levels should vary according to varying degrees of need, and much analytical work is focused on ensuring that appropriate resources relative to need are distributed across the country (Judge and Mays, 1994). Clinical practice also varies, and some of this variation may be avoidable (Bevan and Devlin, 1994), although any dynamic system, such as a market, will inevitably display variations that are the result of innovation and competition.

But what if services are removed from NHS provision altogether in some areas but not in others, such as certain cosmetic and infertility treatments, and with little or no reference to the existence or otherwise of a demand for the service (Redmayne and Klein, 1993)? The prospect then arises of two individuals with precisely the same condition in two different regions of the country, one with access to a service for treating that condition and the other with no access. The only difference between the two individuals is their place of residence. This, on the face of it, offends a sense of 'territorial' justice.

Such local variation might be defended on the grounds that it is simply the proper operation of decentralised decision-making, sensitive to the needs and priorities of different areas. For example, the area without infertility treatment might argue that it has greater needs in other service areas. There are two comments to make here. First, if one area of the country has demonstrably greater health needs than another, then, as noted above, this situation should be (and is) addressed by national rules about the allocation of purchasing power to local areas. Second, even if the specification of *levels* of service for levels of need is an appropriate decision to be made locally, this does not imply that *availability* of service should also be a matter for local judgement, particularly in situations where a need clearly exists to some extent (nobody claims that there are large areas of the country with *no* infertile couples, for example). The non-existence of a service in some areas, coupled with some degree of service in others, is a highly visible form of inequity which promotes a sense of uncertainty about what the NHS is supposed to provide. In such a context, there is a strong case for overriding local discretion.

The point has been made most commonly by those writing with reference to continuing and long-term care:

> *Fair access to health and social care resources in different areas is more than simply a matter of administrative neatness. NHS care is generally free at the point of use, whereas local authority provision and the fee subsidy to residential care of elderly people are both usually means tested. It is patently inequitable if where a person lives dictates whether free or means-tested care becomes available to them.* (Judge and Mays, 1994, p. 1366)

The second reason for specifying more clearly where the boundary of NHS provision lies is more general. There is a growing concern that the users of the NHS are losing a shared, collective understanding of what the NHS is required to provide. This is not just true for a small number of cosmetic procedures in the acute sector, but applies across the continuing and primary care fields as well. Cases brought to the health service commissioner have revealed how health authorities have been refusing to finance the treatment of some individuals in need of long-term care on inappropriate grounds (A. Harrison, 1992 and 1993). Though not new, the issue, in fundamental terms, is this: 'Should those in need of continuing nursing care no longer be entitled to free NHS services and have to bear the burden of payment or be means-tested?' (Whitehead, 1994, p. 1287).

Furthermore, cases brought to the local authority commissioner have shown local government authorities acting in similar ways with regard to decisions as to whether or not to charge for support services for elderly people (A. Harrison, 1992). In the family health service arena, most services apart from the GP consultation itself are now at best subsidised, with many – such as the provision of eye checks and most dental treatment – seeming to disappear from universal provision of any kind.

There is no reason to believe that all these services should automatically be provided free to all – decisions not to provide or to charge for services may be entirely defensible. But the absence of clarity as to what can be expected from the NHS under which circumstances is generating concern and may be undermining a rather more fundamental aspect of the NHS: what Nye Bevan referred to as 'tranquillity'. As argued in the previous chapter, the point of modern health care systems such as the NHS is only in part about prevention and cure – both of which are limited in their effectiveness. It is also about public reassurance, and it is this reassurance which is being undermined by uncertainty. As Christine Hancock put it at a Royal College of Nursing conference:

> *Nobody any longer has confidence in what the NHS would do for them within the limit of its budget … Let's have some core statements about what we can expect of the British Health Service … A list of core values would help to clarify whether there were things the NHS could not afford to do.* (Quoted by Brindle, 1994)

At least some of these core values must relate to the principles on which decisions are made to allocate limited resources to one patient rather than another – the subject of Chapter 5. But they also relate to the boundary between the range of services universally provided by the NHS, and those provided by other agencies or by private finance. A need to start clarifying the boundary is accepted by many researchers, whether it be in the context of purchasing health authorities:

> *…the definition of 'medical need' is itself contentious … purchasers will find themselves dragged increasingly into the process of defining it, in collaboration with the medical profession, however reluctant they may be to move in this direction.* (Redmayne, Klein and Day, 1993, p. 35)

or the analysis of waiting lists:

> *There may be argument about the inequity, divisiveness and practical difficulty of defining those conditions which are and are not eligible for free*

> treatment by the NHS, and argument might be heated. Yet such argument is an essential preliminary to the task of making explicit the limits to potential provision. (Frankel and West, 1993, p. 129)

This chapter will review the possibilities for addressing these concerns.

Conventional approaches to specifying a 'package'

The first two approaches discussed in this chapter – limiting services to those which are effective or cost-effective – have been widely discussed in the literature and will not be dwelt on at length here. However, it is important to distinguish these approaches from the one that follows, since they are quite different in their underlying rationale.

Restricting services to those which are effective

This chapter is largely concerned with principles in the rationing of health care and, in principle, restricting services to those which are effective should be uncontroversial. How could one argue for the positive retention of a procedure which does no good, or even positively does harm? In fact, it could be argued that this is not really rationing at all, since if a medical intervention is of no benefit whatsoever, then no-one is being denied something that they need. But even if the principle is largely uncontroversial, the strategy is unlikely to solve the problem of rationing on its own, and has severe problems in terms of implementation (Bevan and Devlin, 1994; Hunter, 1994).

However, even assuming a consensus on principle is perhaps unwise. Undertaking a procedure which does not improve health may improve well-being in other ways. In other words, what economists have called 'process utility' can be important – in this case, being 'cared for' is valued by a patient even if the treatment is not improving health, *per se*. An over-zealous preoccupation with 'health' as the only relevant output of the NHS has been criticised (Mooney, 1994), and lies behind some of the concerns of the incrementalists identified in Chapter 3. As was argued previously, if what people really value is reassurance, or community, or 'fairness', then rigorous exclusion on scientific grounds of all procedures which do not produce 'health' may prove unpopular, not to say difficult to implement.

Practical difficulties, though, are likely to prove the most serious obstacle to this approach 'solving' the problem of rationing. Procedures which are ineffective for most people may be effective for a few, and this means that the number of procedures which could be excluded altogether, on the basis that they do *no good to anyone*, is likely to be very small in practice.

The central problem is that, although the strategy appears to be focused on services, it is actually concerned with the average effect on people. To say a service is ineffective is really saying that trials have shown that, on average, the procedure has a negligible or even negative effect on a group of people. Individuals within that group, however – the human race being highly heterogeneous – may still benefit. Partly because of this, the medical profession is likely to resist strategies which it sees as merely geared toward containing costs, while restricting their clinical freedom to choose the best treatment for the individual patient with whom they are concerned. All this is not to reject the approach outright, merely to emphasise that the prospect for restricting the number of services will be limited, as the New Zealand reformers discovered (Cooper, 1995).

Restricting services to those which are cost-effective

The second of the conventional approaches involves restricting the menu with reference to cost-effectiveness. Given a limited budget, services should be ranked according to their relative cost-effectiveness; then, starting with the most cost-effective procedure, the services should be included in the package one-by-one until the budget runs out. By restricting services to those which are the most cost-effective, the health benefit to be gained from a limited budget can be maximised. This is the original strategy adopted by the State of Oregon – although later much modified – and is the subject of a vast literature (see for example, Fox and Leichter, 1991; Strosberg *et al.*, 1992; Kitzhaber, 1995).[2]

The first point to note is that, unlike limiting the package with reference to effectiveness alone, where the final range of services is independent of

---

2. Another, rather more subtle, variant on the cost-effectiveness approach has been suggested by Ronald Dworkin, with the focus on what an individual would consider as cost-effective for themselves. He suggests a 'prudent insurance principle' to guide what is included in a public health care package. It sets up a thought experiment based on what people would insure against under fair circumstances and with full knowledge of costs and benefits; as such, though, it remains a derivative of cost-effectiveness approaches, but based in contractarian political philosophy (see Dworkin, 1994 for a full discussion).

any other considerations, here 'where the line is drawn' will always be linked to the size of the budget. This will, in turn, always be politically contentious. The approach does not achieve any lasting consensus about the range of services to be included, even if the principle underlying it is agreed upon. The second point is that exactly the same problem which bedevils the effectiveness approach recurs for cost-effectiveness – the assessment of relative cost-effectiveness is based on the calculation of average scores from groups of people. Some treatments which might be excluded from a package of health care could be highly cost-effective for certain individuals. Again, the problem derives from an attempt to conceptualise exclusions in terms of *services* when what is being measured is the *effects* of services on people who are highly heterogeneous.

The political difficulties of explicitly excluding services from the NHS on the basis of cost were discussed earlier in this report. It may be necessary, and ethically defensible, for the medical profession, and others, to take cost into account when making decisions regarding the allocation of scarce resources. This is entirely different from an *ex ante* exclusion of the service from NHS provision altogether. Any policy which excluded services on the basis of cost is certain, at the very least, to cause substantial political controversy and professional resistance.

The problem of heterogeneity

Both of these strategies run up against the problem of the heterogeneous nature of the effects of health services. With reference to the first strategy, it is not going to be easy to exclude a significant number of services purely on grounds of ineffectiveness. It should be emphasised, however, that where a consensus does emerge that certain services are genuinely of no benefit to anyone, then their exclusion on a national basis may be justified. But until a national consensus is demonstrated, there seems little option other than to leave decisions to individual clinicians. The second strategy is even more contentious: *ex ante* exclusions on the basis of cost are difficult to defend in principle, awkward to implement in practice and, from a political perspective, quite probably impossible to undertake, in this country at least.[3]

---

3. This is not to say that it cannot be done. The State of Oregon achieved it, but, it could be argued, the alternative for Oregonians – significant numbers of uninsured poor people – was worse. The UK does not start from this position.

Effectiveness and cost are more properly discussed in terms of their appropriateness as criteria for discriminating between people, and are analysed as such in Chapter 5. But there remains a legitimate question: what is the range of services which is *relevant* to NHS activity? Is everything which is of benefit, and which is within the competence of the NHS and its employees to provide, relevant to the goals of the NHS? In the remainder of this chapter a third approach to defining the range or 'menu' of services will be presented. It focuses on the characteristics of services themselves, rather than the quantification of their effects on people.

The need for a new approach

Many of the services discussed earlier – long-term nursing care, fertility treatment, dentistry and cosmetic procedures – are not generally considered to be ineffective. Neither are they particularly costly, at least not when compared with many procedures in the acute sector. Why, then, do they not appear to be part of regular NHS provision?

The approach to answering this question presented below involves 'identifying services which do not seem to belong in a system of health care which is publicly financed' (Bevan and Devlin, 1994, p. 2). Bevan and Devlin do not delve any deeper, however, concluding immediately that 'this approach generates a list of exclusions which is disappointingly small in terms of relieving pressure on NHS resources' (ibid., 1994). This, however, misses the point: an appropriate policy for specifying the range of NHS services should not just ease the pressure on financing, but should clarify what can be expected from the NHS and promote equity in the range of available services across the country. Furthermore, as we have seen, the issues go far wider than merely tattoo removal and infertility treatment. In particular, the division of responsibilities for long-term care is an issue growing in salience, and with consequences for large amounts of public money. Suggestions for drawing a boundary around what the NHS should do have also been made in this context:

> *There is a conceptually simple way in which this problem could be solved. If the NHS became responsible only for investigation, diagnoses, treatment and rehabilitation, and long-term care of all forms in the community or institution became the responsibility of the [putative] Community Agency,*

> the boundaries of the two agencies could be unambiguously defined.
> (Grimley Evans, quoted in A. Harrison, 1993, p. 30)

Whether or not this is true, it begs the question of finance. As matters stand, NHS care is free, whereas various forms of long-term and social care are not. What are the salient features of long-term care that lead society increasingly to charge for its provision? What, indeed, have tattoo removal and nursing care got in common that they are increasingly excluded from universal provision?

Further examples abound. Eye tests might also seem to lie clearly within the health care arena, but now such tests are subsidised for only a proportion of the population. General dentistry is universally subsidised, but to such a small proportion of its real cost that to many it must appear as though it has been effectively excluded from the NHS. The already confused picture is complicated by the number of agencies involved, notably local authorities who have a large measure of discretion as to whether or not they provide certain 'support' services free.

'Excluded' services in the USA and UK

The NHS is not the only health care system which has attempted to define its boundaries. As we have seen, New Zealand and Holland investigated the possibilities, but have not managed to outline specific services. However, President Clinton's ill-fated Health Security Act did specifically state included and excluded services; those excluded are listed in Table 2. Compared with the situation in the UK, its drafters had the advantage of engaging in a comprehensive review of a health care system rather than undertaking administrative changes to an existing one, and such a context makes it relatively easy to reflect on what a 'comprehensive' health care package should be. Nevertheless, the list demonstrates the possibilities for approaching reform of this kind.

Interestingly, there is no explicit analysis of how the items listed in Table 2 were selected. Many of the items might intuitively appear appropriate for exclusion from a universal health care system, but unless there were robust reasons for the list it might have proved hard to defend if the Act had become law. Many might argue that infertility services, for example,

Table 2 Clinton's exclusions

- Custodial care (except in the case of hospice care)
- Cosmetic surgery (other than to correct congenital anomalies or following an accident or disease)
- Hearing aids
- Eyeglasses and contact lenses for individuals 18 years of age and older
- *In vitro* fertilisation services
- Sex change and related services
- Private duty nursing
- Personal comfort items (except in the case of hospice care)
- Orthodontol and other dental procedures other than those described elsewhere in the Act (NB: the Act *included* most common dental procedures)

The Act also excludes those 'items or services that are not medically necessary or appropriate' as regulated by a new National Health Board.[4]

Source: Health Security Act 1993, Library of Congress, Washington; see also Fuchs and Merlis (1993)

should be included as a health care service, and it seems inadvisable not to offer any sort of rationale for their exclusion.

Nevertheless, the US proposals at least offered clarity: no-one could have been in any doubt about the range of services to which they were entitled, and the range of those to which they were not. In contrast, the UK has no such list. The legislation on which NHS provision is now based – the National Health Service Act 1977 – only places a duty on the Secretary of State to provide health services to a 'reasonable' level, and makes only a few specific inclusions, such as maternity services – in that case presumably so as to avoid any confusion as to whether childbirth should be counted as warranting 'health care'.

A mixture of local health authority (and occasionally local government) decisions, coupled with national rules on charging and excluded medicines, has resulted in a peculiarly incoherent distribution of services between universal and non-universal provision. Table 3 represents this split with the solid line, and also represents the range of costs to users at the point of use both on the universal and non-universal sides of the line.

---

4. This seems to allow for the exclusion of services on the basis of ineffectiveness or cost-ineffectiveness – what the Act termed 'inappropriate' care; see, for example, Working Group Report to Director of Research & Development, 1993.

Table 3 Range of costs to users of various health-related services

Broad service categories	Nature of cost to service user			
	Universal state provision		Residual state provision	No state provision
	'Free'[1]	Access & time costs	Subsidised price to all (with additional means tests)	Subsidised price to some (with means tests)	Market price only
Acute and 'community' services	Emergencies	Consultations, elective surgery, out-patients, 'community' services, etc.	–	–	Cosmetic and infertility services [2]
Continuing care services	–	Long-term 'medical' care [2]	Aids and appliances.[2] Day, domiciliary and respite services [2]	Long-term 'non-medical' residential or nursing care	–
Family health services	–	GP consultation	Prescribed drugs, dental care	Eye tests/prescriptions, spectacles, hearing aids, some self-care medication	'Medicines' on limited list (not available for NHS prescription)

1 'Free' is placed in inverted commas because it is recognised that even emergencies are subject to time costs, and individuals do not always get immediate treatment even after arriving at hospital.

2 Depending on area. Although long-term, or continuing, medical care is an NHS responsibility under the 1977 Act, some health authorities have been accused of running down their long-stay bed capacity, effectively evading a commitment to continuing care.

Emergencies are the only services which approach genuine 'free' state at the point of use: the individual (normally) suffers a very short waiting time and ambulance provision is free and fast. The vast majority of NHS services, however, are subject to time costs – waiting lists and GP appointments – or access costs – travel is not generally free for elective procedures or outpatient services. Nevertheless, these two categories of costs reflect what is generally understood to be free NHS provision.

However, the next category of cost – subsidised price to all – is also universal in nature since no-one is excluded from at least a partial subsidy, although the degree of subsidy does vary according to the user's contingency. So, for both prescribed drugs and dental treatment, certain groups of users – for example, elderly people, pregnant women and those on low incomes – are subsidised such that the money cost to them is zero.

To the right of the solid line, provision is no longer universal, since a large proportion of the population must pay the market price – or, as is the case with certain of the cheaper drugs, the subsidy for all is insufficient to provide an incentive to prescribe. GPs now regularly advise an 'over-the-counter' purchase where appropriate for those not exempt from prescription charges for medicines costing less than the current charge. The final column – market price only – relates to those health-related services which are not subject to any government intervention. This is a relatively small category since, as one would expect, any service related in any way to health or well-being is typically subsidised to some degree to ensure that those on low incomes are not unfairly prevented from benefiting. However, as we have seen, certain acute services in some areas are now excluded, and the 'limited list' of medication which can no longer be prescribed on the NHS grows yearly.

It is not at all obvious why the configuration of services in Table 3 is as it is in the UK. Studies of the provision of *in vitro* fertilisation have revealed that health authorities have a number of different reasons for both including and excluding infertility services, but with little consistency from one authority to another (Klein and Redmayne, 1993). Health authorities also appear unsure of their responsibilities with regard to long-term care – something which recent guidance from the Department of Health has attempted to clarify (Department of Health, 1995). The 1977 Act requires the provision of some 'after-care', where 'appropriate', but there was a suspicion that some health authorities were effectively removing their long-stay bed availability. And the health ombudsman has ruled that a health authority has a duty to provide care at no cost to the patient where he or she needs 'sustained nursing care for the rest of her life' (quoted in A. Harrison, 1992, p. 39). When is nursing care 'medically necessary'; where does 'nursing' care end and 'social' care begin? And even if residential care is clearly non-medical, why is the state not providing a universal service when many would see the forms of care in residential homes as every bit as necessary as, for example, hip replacements? The picture is equally confused with respect to domiciliary, respite and day care services provided by local authorities.

Perhaps the rationale for non-universal provision is most obscure in the case of some family health services. Eye tests, spectacles and hearing aids, and some cheap medicines, are now only subsidised to a proportion of the population. Dental treatment is only subsidised for a small proportion of the real cost. And yet these services would seem intuitively to lie squarely within the health care field, and therefore be prime candidates for universal provision.

Rationale for universal provision: health care as a 'special' service

Trying to explain why provision is organised in the way it is requires a careful historical analysis of how policy has developed, paying particular attention to the political circumstances and context in which those changes took place. Such an investigation is not the purpose of this analysis. We wish to set out a coherent framework for deciding what should be the range of services on offer from the NHS. This may also inform our understanding of the historical development of the current provision, but it is not our central aim.

The central feature of our approach is to investigate, from first principles, what it is about health care which makes it 'special', marking it out from other goods and services. The first point to note is that the demand for health care is a derived demand for health: the important aspects of the delivery of health care relate to the nature of health and ill health. In this book we refer in general to health care but in this chapter reference will need to be made to health. The two concepts are not being confused but their close relationship is important to the following discussion.

Economists and moral philosophers have both made their quite different contributions to our understanding of the special nature of health care. The special economic nature of the health care industry was first subjected to systematic and rigorous analysis 30 years ago in a seminal article by Arrow (1963). There he isolated uncertainty as the key characteristic of the demand for health care which made its efficient exchange in private markets problematic. Two elements of uncertainty – unpredictability and information imbalance – together contributed to its difficulties.

Arrow was not interested in the moral aspects of health care delivery; that was the domain of moral philosophers. They had their own reasons for suspecting that the market was an inappropriate medium for health care delivery, namely that it resulted in an unfair distribution of health services (see, for example, Daniels, 1985; Churchill, 1987; Rhodes, 1992, for detailed examinations of just allocations of health care). The precise justification for this unfairness varies from author to author: Daniels, for example, emphasises how ill health impairs an individual's share of the 'normal opportunity range for his society ... individuals have a *fundamental* interest in protecting that share' (1985, p. 57, emphasis added). But a common factor in philosophical analyses of health care is some sense of its fundamental importance.

It is worth reflecting on these sources of market failure (unpredictability; information imbalance; and fundamental importance) in turn.

Unpredictability and information imbalance – inefficient markets

Ill health is inherently unpredictable: if we knew when we were going to fall ill or have an accident we could provide for the consequences. As it is, like other unpredictable eventualities, the typical response for all those other than risk-seekers is to pay a third party to bear the risk – take out insurance. Unpredictability is obviously a widespread phenomenon and so cannot on its own explain health care's special nature. However, health care is also subject to extreme information imbalances: we do not as a rule know the nature of what is wrong with us nor how to return to good health. The classic assumption of the perfect competition model of economic exchange – that by and large the individual is the best judge of what is in his or her best interests – does not hold for the demand for health care.

These two characteristics together make health care extremely problematic for economic exchange. Insurance markets do not work well under such conditions. The reasons have been analysed at length elsewhere (see, for example, Cullis and West, 1979; Mooney, 1986; and McGuire *et al.*, 1988). In summary, patients do not know what is in their best interests, and rely on the medical profession to make the choices for them; doctors, in turn, have an incentive to supply as much treatment as possible because a third party pays. The result is a problem of oversupply and escalating costs. This is compounded by incentives for patients not to reveal the true nature of their risk factors – consequently, when risks are pooled, low-risk individuals will typically pay premiums which are higher than their expected benefit. Such individuals may decide not to insure at all when in principle there are welfare gains from so doing – a problem known as adverse selection.

The problems associated with the economic exchange of health care services via insurance markets are a good deal more complex than this, and the demand for health care has other characteristics which make matters even more problematic. But for our purposes it is sufficient to summarise the position as conditions of unpredictability and information imbalance leading to a combination of overprovision for some and no provision for others. This debate, after Arrow's initial contribution, was often conducted in *a priori* terms, drawing on economic theory to predict how the market would, or would not, fail. In the 1970s Culyer argued that ultimately the truth or otherwise of such predictions could only be established with reference to empirical evidence (Culyer, 1971). It is interesting to note that the USA, the only developed country genuinely to 'experiment' with a free market in health care insurance as the principal means of finance, persistently suffered from escalating costs and non-insurance on a scale experienced nowhere else.

Fundamental importance – inequitable markets

The fact that health is fundamental to most other forms of satisfaction or pleasure is a reasonably uncontroversial proposition. This in itself provides health care with a certain moral importance: it is an insufficient reason that someone should not be able to afford health care for them to be denied it. Furthermore, the fact that, in general, we are not responsible for our ill health, or at least only partially responsible, gives further weight to the argument that we should not be forced to face the, possibly severe, consequences of eventualities beyond our control.

It could be argued, however, that although we are not responsible for our ill health, we are responsible for not insuring against the consequences, if we have sufficient resources. So, as long as adequate income transfer policies are implemented so that health care insurance is within financial reach of everyone, the state's obligation on equity grounds has been discharged. But this option has not satisfied most developed nations: the state has typically taken responsibility for ensuring that some form of insurance is taken out by everyone – there is an element of compulsion – or that there is a free service such as the NHS. The problem of inequitable markets is therefore complicated by the fact that typically governments act with a degree of paternalism: they are not satisfied that all individuals will act in their own best interests. Nevertheless, it is clearly linked to the idea that health is fundamentally important, and so issues related to misjudging one's own interest are included under this heading.

In any event, free markets typically produce gross inequities in access to health care. Low-income groups will often resist the purchase of insurance in favour of more immediate necessities such as food, clothing and shelter. The problem of adverse selection means that many better-off individuals will also fail to insure, and when ill health strikes, the costs of treatment will typically be beyond the means of all but the richest of those without insurance. The distribution of health and health care will be unjust without government intervention. While this last assertion is not universally accepted, even the USA, as we have seen, has recently attempted to implement a health care system in which everyone has guaranteed access.

Health care – a special service

It is important to note that these three characteristics taken together give health care its special nature and should encourage governments to become involved in its universal provision or regulation. Simply displaying unpredictability and information imbalance is insufficient reason in itself. The insurance market for car repairs after a serious accident provides a case in point. Accidents are by their nature unpredictable, and we know very little about what is needed to repair a badly damaged car; breakdowns often occur without an accident being involved, and it may not be at all clear what has gone wrong; there may be a mechanical fault without our being aware of it; and so on. All these situations are similar in terms of information imbalance to ill health. There is, in all likelihood, a danger of over-provision of car repair work in private markets. But this does not necessarily warrant state intervention, as car repair work would not generally be considered sufficiently important to justify the extra taxation and limitations on personal freedom which that intervention would entail.

Fundamental importance on its own is not enough either. Food is obviously fundamental to our very existence, and yet there is no 'national food service'. The reason is that the need for food is predictable and there is little information imbalance; nor is there perceived to be a problem of people not knowing their own best interests. The problem of fundamental importance, therefore, can be overcome simply by income transfers to those who would otherwise have insufficient money to feed themselves. There is no need for universal provision.

Health care and heterogeneity

These three characteristics – unpredictability, information imbalance and fundamental importance – describe or define health care's special nature as if it were a homogeneous good. Indeed, all the analyses outlined above which discussed the moral and economic problems with health care did the same. But, as we have seen, health care services are anything but homogeneous and the three characteristics apply to most, but not all, of what might be termed health-related services.

Analysing the characteristics of health care services

How do the services in Table 3 match up to these criteria? Long-term residential care, for example, is quite clearly of fundamental importance, but it is less clear that it satisfies the criterion of information imbalance. Certainly, there will be those elderly frail or chronically ill people who will find it difficult to exercise the faculties necessary to make informed choices in a market context. But they would also presumably find it difficult successfully to exercise choice informed with good information about *most* goods and services; long-term care provision may not be qualitatively different in this specific sense. Many people in need of long-term residential care may be quite well informed, indeed better informed than anyone else, as to the nature of care they need. The fundamental importance of long-term care, assuming this is agreed, is not sufficient reason necessarily to provide a universal service when equity concerns can be addressed via income transfers.[5]

Long-term *nursing* care presents a more difficult case. Nursing care is not easy to define or specify: it includes a whole range of activities stretching from those relating to simple acts of caring, to those which we might ordinarily think of as relatively complex medical interventions (Beardshaw and Robinson, 1990). So, if a typical nursing home involves care and support which are of a fairly routine kind – help with 'feeding, bathing, dressing and movement; giving drugs and other treatments; and talking to, reassuring and informing patients and their families' (ibid., p. 7) – then the criteria do not seem to apply. Long-term nursing care of this kind should not be provided on a universal basis by the NHS.

However, there are other forms of need for nursing services. In 1991 a man was discharged from hospital while still in need of intensive nursing care after suffering a brain haemorrhage. He will be highly dependent for the rest of his life (see A. Harrison, 1994, pp. 23–4, for a summary of the case).

---

5. A situation where an individual suffers from some form of mental incapacity – handicap, illness, dementia, etc. – presents a special case which deserves more analysis than can be provided here. These individuals clearly suffer from severe information imbalance by definition of their condition; it may be that they automatically deserve universal provision on this basis alone. On the other hand, if they have sufficient financial means, it may be reasonable to encourage an advocate – family member or other agent – to make decisions on their behalf, depending on the form of care necessary.

The health authority refused to pay for nursing home care, on the basis that this form of continuing care was not an NHS responsibility. The man's wife complained to the Health Service Commissioner, who upheld the complaint. The patient was highly dependent, and the form of care he required would almost certainly satisfy the criteria.

Nursing care cannot easily be categorised: although routine nursing home care should not be provided universally, on our criteria there *is* a need for certain forms of intensive nursing to be provided on this basis. The criteria outlined in this chapter could guide the selection of individuals for whom NHS care is appropriate; they might also point to a need for increased provision of NHS nursing homes.

Other services are less difficult from an analytical viewpoint. The provision of hearing aids and spectacles also fail clearly to display the special characteristics. Again, good sight and hearing may be of fundamental importance (although to the many blind and deaf individuals this may in itself be something of an exaggeration), but it is not clear that there is significant information imbalance or uncertainty. And cosmetic surgery is often singled out for removal from NHS provision and here, again, the criteria support such a policy. Information balance and uncertainty are not severe (we are not considering reconstructive surgery, merely elective procedures for aesthetic purposes); in fact, the recipient of cosmetic procedures is the best person to judge their 'success'.

There is a distinction to be made between having good knowledge of the techniques of surgery, spectacle manufacture or nursing good practice, which most of us clearly do not have, and understanding what is amiss, what is broadly speaking necessary to put it right, and whether we can be confident that we have got what we need after the service has been provided – which most of us do in the services analysed above. After all, we have very little knowledge or information about how a vast range of goods and services are provided for us, but this does not prevent us from being the best judge of whether they satisfy our wants, needs or desires. This applies equally to goods of fundamental importance such as food, clothing and shelter. The fact that we know little of the techniques of the manufacture of clothing, or how in scientific terms food nourishes us, does not lead us to demand universal provision.

So far, we have analysed those interventions which the criteria would suggest are not relevant to NHS provision. However, other interventions which our earlier analysis indicated were in danger of being excluded from NHS provision, do seem to satisfy the criteria. For example, curative dentistry, including procedures such as fillings, is subject to substantial information imbalance and uncertainty: very often the need for a filling, and its operation, is undertaken without our having any sensation of ill-effects. We are not sufficiently competent to judge the necessity or success of the procedure. And a toothache can certainly seem of fundamental importance – at least while it lasts!

Similarly, sight check-ups, to the extent that they screen for more serious medical complaints such as diabetes, glaucoma and forms of ocular cancer, are also subject to information imbalances: we are unaware of the full range of benefits to be gained from a check-up. Dental checks provide a similar service in the early diagnosis of potentially expensive conditions. These procedures are essentially concerned with screening for future ill health, and there will be questions to resolve about their cost-effectiveness for various categories of individual. However, if there is agreed to be a cost-effective preventive element, then these checks should be part of NHS provision.

In vitro fertilisation provides another test for the usefulness of the criteria. We seem to have good information about the nature of the problem – difficulty in conceiving a child. We also have some knowledge about whether the treatment has worked or not. Is this not then a good case for advising that the service be left to private market transactions? We may even bolster the case by arguing that the condition of fundamental importance is not satisfied either: nobody is suffering physically, let alone dying.

However, this does not seem persuasive on closer reflection. We do not have good information on the nature of the problem in clinical terms. We have to take the advice of a clinician as to the nature of the dysfunction and the likelihood of remedies to succeed. If fertilisation is not achieved we are in no position other than to accept the physician's advice as to the likely efficacy of further attempts; if fertilisation is achieved we must accept assurances that this was the direct result of the treatment. Although there may be some scope for shopping around, unlike many medical complaints, with such information imbalances it will be difficult to make comparisons. In a private market, particularly with insurance cover, there will be incentives to over-provide: where the marginal benefit in terms of probability of success is less than the marginal cost in terms of extra insurance premiums or out-of-pocket payments. And is not the inability to have a child of fundamental importance? The psychological stress alone may be far more disabling than many physical complaints.

The need for judgement

The principle, therefore, can be stated thus: that services included under the aegis of the NHS and thus provided on a universal basis should display characteristics of uncertainty, information imbalance and fundamental importance. However, the analysis of the examples above has shown that the criteria do not provide a definitive methodology for deciding what should constitute the range of NHS services. In other words, there will remain a need for judgement.

However, this is only to be expected. No principle can hope to specify action so precisely that the need for further thought and judgement is unnecessary. In this context, there will always be a need to decide to what extent the criteria apply. Table 4 provides our judgement of some services which, according to the criteria, should not be part of NHS provision, as well as some examples of services which seem to drifting out of the NHS, but which should remain inside. These follow directly from the discussion above; it is not an exhaustive list, but provides an indication of the implications of the approach.

This approach does not obviate the need to assess individual cases, particularly where an individual moves from one service category to another. For example, an elderly person who has a fall and needs acute care may subsequently need either continuing medical care or residential care. A clinical judgement will inevitably need to be made about the form of care which becomes necessary, and this will determine whether universal NHS care continues or whether other forms of care begin. It is noteworthy that recent Department of Health guidance asserts that continuing medical care – including palliative, in-patient, respite and specialist care for those in nursing or residential homes – must be made available on the NHS by virtue of its 'complexity or intensity' (Department of Health, 1995, p.24).

Table 4 Examples of services which should be 'outside' NHS responsibilities, and those which should be 'inside'

'Out'	'In'
• Residential care for elderly people	• Continuing medical care
• Routine nursing home care for elderly people	• Medical or specialist nursing services for those in residential care
• Cosmetic dental treatment; provision of spectacles and hearing aids	• Curative dental treatment (including restorative work such as fillings); preventative dental and sight check-ups
• Cosmetic surgery (enhancement)	• Cosmetic surgery (reconstructive)
• Medicines for non-complex conditions (e.g. headaches, hay fever)	• Fertility treatments

This is not dissimilar to the criteria of information imbalance. The government does not, of course, apply this approach systematically across the whole spectrum of health-related services.

Services need to be carefully and tightly defined for this approach to be of use: it is no good vaguely specifying long-term care, dentistry or whatever. Furthermore, the services themselves are of interest, not the locus of their delivery: occasional specialist nursing care for instance, which is required in a residential home, should be provided on a universal basis. However, the general point is that fundamental importance, information imbalance and unpredictability vary from one service to another, not between individuals in receipt of the service. In other words, there are *qualitative* differences between services which are reflected in the fact that we assign definitional categories to them. This allows services to be specified on the basis of these criteria without running into the difficulties with heterogeneity associated with similar attempts based on cost and effectiveness.

Conclusion: what should be done?

The boundary between what the NHS does and what other agencies do, or what individuals should do for themselves, is at present developing on an *ad hoc* case-law basis, and this cannot promote a sense of geographical equity, nor a clear, shared understanding of what the NHS should provide. Further debate and analysis are required before an approach such as that described above could be implemented. But what is perhaps most interesting is that none of the countries mentioned at the beginning of this chapter has managed successfully to draw up an agreed package with any degree of precision. In Holland, a Government Committee advised that health services must be 'necessary, effective, efficient and cannot be left to the individual's responsibility' (van de Ven, 1995) if they were to be included in a basic health care package, but services are not specified. In New Zealand, as we saw at the beginning of this chapter, those attempting to specify a package concluded that it was impossible to defend excluding *any* service currently provided. The analysis of this chapter suggests that their attempts would have been helped by distinguishing exclusions on effectiveness or cost-effectiveness grounds from exclusions related to criteria which give health care its 'special' nature.

Attempting to exclude services *ex ante* on the basis of (lack of) effectiveness or cost-effectiveness will inevitably be hampered by the heterogeneous nature of health care. One may be able to conceive of a service as a homogeneous entity, but this does not imply that its effect on individual patients will be. Not only is health care heterogeneous, but so are individual health care interventions.

The heterogeneous nature of health care should also alert us to the fact that everything which could provide benefit, and which is within the capability of health care professionals to provide, is not equally appropriate for universal provision. There is a case for a specific catalogue of NHS services defined at national level, together with some exclusions along the lines of the Clinton Act. All purchasing authorities would be required to provide all the services thereby specified, although the level of service provision would remain a matter for local discretion. This might at least start to bring some consistency and coherence to the present uncertainty and piecemeal development of policy. Not everything can always be on the menu; we need to start devising ways of clarifying what might be left off.

Chapter 5

Principles of rationing: choosing between people

Suppose that, following the principles of Chapter 4, it has been decided that a given package of health care services has the characteristics – uncertainty, information imbalance, fundamental importance – that mean they should be provided free at the point of use. Given that, as with anything provided free, the demand for these services is likely to exceed the available provision, there remains the problem of rationing the services between competing users: between patients. How should patients be prioritised? Can this be done in a rational manner? What principles should guide the rationing decisions? It is to these questions that this chapter is addressed.

Chapter 4 argued that discriminating between treatments to be provided free at the point of use and other services required the identification of certain characteristics of the treatments concerned. The parallel to this in the patient case is to examine the characteristics of *patients* to see whether those characteristics offer a basis for discrimination between people. Obviously, some of those characteristics would relate to patients' immediate need for treatment: how ill they were, how effective the treatment was likely to be in their case, and so on. However, as was illustrated earlier, there are many situations where the rationing decision has been influenced by characteristics of patients that were not to do with their immediate need, such as their age or their smoking habits. So in what follows we consider both need-related characteristics and characteristics unrelated to need as possible influences on the rationing decision.

Need-related characteristics

In a broad sense, need has to be a necessary characteristic of any patient who is to be offered treatment. There is no point in giving treatment to someone who does not need it. However, this begs the question as to how need should be defined, and how patients with different types of need should be prioritised. Now, 'need' is a slippery concept and there have been many attempts to pin it down (see, for instance, Williams, 1978; Culyer, 1995). We do not want to enter that debate here; instead we concentrate simply on two possible interpretations of the term, either of which could be used to affect the rationing decision.

The first interpretation defines need purely in terms of the extent of illness: that is, the more ill a patient is, the more needy she is and the higher priority she should be given. On this interpretation, those in greatest need of health care are those who are the most ill, or, put another way, those who have the largest health 'deficit'. Rationing based on this conception of need would give more health care to those with the larger health deficit.

One version of this principle is the 'rescue principle' (as formulated, and attacked, by Dworkin, 1994) whereby everything should be sacrificed to preserve life. The rescue principle is often invoked when an identified individual is in danger of dying: a child in need of a liver transplant, or a potholer stuck in a cave with a broken leg. Such single cases can absorb very large amounts of resources, but nonetheless frequently acquire top priority for resource allocation, especially if well publicised.

This principle derives from a yet more fundamental principle: that health states should, so far as possible, be equalised. So, if one individual has a greater health deficit than another, then the first individual should have priority of treatment at least until his or her health state is brought up to that of the other. It is thus fundamentally egalitarian in nature. But its appeal is wider than this. To offer an individual the chance of a complete recovery from a life-threatening illness or other event would be valued by many supporters of the NHS, even if that chance was a small one.

Obvious practical problems arise in implementation. How should 'health deficit' be defined for operational purposes? Does it refer to pain or distress? To closeness to death? What about the length of time spent waiting for treatment? Also, there is the practical question as to who determines the degree of health deficit: the clinician, the hospital manager – or the patient herself?

Even if the practical problems could be overcome, rationing according to this characteristic could lead to unacceptable outcomes. For instance, as with its application in the form of the rescue principle, it would imply that someone who is terminally ill (presumably the ultimate health deficit) should receive maximum health care, regardless of the likely outcome of that care. This could result in massive quantities of care being devoted to patients with no realistic chance of recovery; an allocation that is certainly inefficient, and perhaps also inequitable with respect to those who were less ill – in the sense of not being terminally ill – but who could have benefited from the resources concerned had they been employed in a different way.

In fact, it is possible to argue that this method of rationing is one already employed in many medical systems and that it is indeed seriously wasteful. A recent report concluded that too many operations were being undertaken in the NHS to too little effect on those close to death (National Confidential Enquiry into Perioperative Deaths, 1993). In the USA, it has been estimated that the mean Medicare payment for the last year of life was seven times that of the average yearly payment for all Medicare patients, and payments during the last *month* of life constituted 40 per cent of payments during the last year of life (Lubitz and Riley, 1993).

More generally, a serious weakness of the use of this characteristic as a method of rationing health care is that it concentrates solely upon the health of the potential recipient of care and not on the ability of the recipient to benefit from that care. This suggests that it might be more appropriate to interpret the need for care in terms of the likely effectiveness or efficacy of that care or, put another way, in terms of the individual patient's capacity to benefit from care. Under this interpretation, patients in greatest need are those who have the greatest capacity to benefit; hence, the more responsive to treatment a patient is and hence the more effective the treatment, the higher priority she should be given.

Applying these two interpretations of need in many situations will yield the same conclusion. Often those who are suffering most from a particular condition – that is, those who are most ill – are those who respond most successfully to treatment and for whom treatment is most effective. Hence rationing according to degree of illness will be the same as rationing according to effectiveness.

But this will not always be so. For instance, treatment at an early stage of a condition is often more effective than at a later stage when the disease has really taken hold. In such cases should patients at the early stages be prioritised over those at later stages, despite the fact that the latter are suffering more? Or should the extent of patient suffering dominate the decision? The interpretation of need according to capacity to benefit would say yes to the first question and no to the second; the interpretation according to health deficit, the reverse.

A further complication concerns cost. What if it is more costly to treat one patient than another for the same condition? What if, as seems plausible, the more ill patients are, the more expensive they are to treat? What if the more *responsive* patients are more expensive to treat?

Cost and responsiveness considerations can be merged by using the cost-effectiveness of treatment as the patient characteristic for rationing. That is, patients who cost less to achieve a given response to treatment are prioritised over those who cost more. This is the rationale behind the well-known cost-per-QALY procedure for rationing. Here the measure of responsiveness is taken as the number of quality-adjusted-life-years (QALYs) gained from applying a particular procedure to a particular patient; this is divided into the total cost of the procedure to give the cost-per-QALY gained. Patients with low costs-per-QALY are then given priority over those with higher ones.

The advocates of the cost-effectiveness approach to rationing justify it in two ways (Lockwood, 1988; Williams, 1988). First, if the overall aim of a health system is to obtain as much health improvement as possible from limited resources, this is the most efficient way to do it. For, by concentrating on low cost-per-QALY patients, more resources are available for treating more patients and thus more aggregate health gain can be achieved. This seems desirable on the grounds that, other things being equal, it is better to treat more people than less. Second, it seems fundamentally equitable; for it gives each year of life an equal weight, regardless of to whom it accrues.

On the other hand, its claims with respect to equity have been challenged (Harris, 1988). As so often with principles that promote efficiency, its application under some circumstances can produce outcomes that seem intuitively inequitable or unfair. Most obviously, it will discriminate against those patients who, through no fault of their own, need very expensive treatments. As we have seen earlier, this may include those who are extremely ill; hence consistent application of this principle may involve discrimination against the very ill. The upshot of that is that its implementation may be quite compatible with inequality in health outcomes (Culyer, 1988).

It may also result in other, more subtle forms of discrimination. For instance, it is often the case that poor people respond worse to medical treatment than wealthier people with the same condition – because the latter are better fed, live in more salubrious housing, and have superior support systems at home. In that situation, treatment of rich individuals might have a lower cost-per-QALY, or, what is the same thing, a higher health gain (as measured in QALYs) per pound than treatment of poor individuals in the same state of ill health. Now, if individuals are weighted equally in the process of aggregating health gain (that is, a QALY is treated as the same, whether accruing to a poor or a rich individual), then allocating health care on the basis of health gain per pound or cost-per-QALY will result in giving wealthy people priority over poor people; not an outcome that everybody would regard as fair.

Another example of a potentially unfair outcome resulting from the application of this rationing procedure with equal weighting of individuals, concerns elderly people. If effectiveness or health gain is measured by QALYs, for instance, or indeed by any measure that involves years of life gained by treatment, this is likely to discriminate in favour of younger people. A life-saving treatment given to a baby, for example, would result in a larger number of life-years gained than if the same treatment were given at the same cost to a 60-year old (or a 40- or a 20-year old). Hence, the cost-per-QALY would be lower for the baby than the older individuals and the baby would be prioritised. More generally, other things being equal, life-expectancy would dominate rationing procedures and this might not be universally regarded as fair.

Finally, for life-threatening diseases, this rationing characteristic with equal individual weights could discriminate against disabled persons –

again especially if QALYs or related measures of the quality of life were used to measure capacity to benefit, and QALYs are weighted equally regardless of to whom they accrue. Other things being equal, the QALY measurement procedure attributes fewer QALYs to disabled people than able-bodied persons of the same overall life-expectancy. Hence treating a disabled person for a life-threatening disease that was not related to her disability would generate fewer QALYs than the same treatment given to an able-bodied person with the same disease. The result would be a higher cost-per-QALY and therefore a lower priority for the disabled patient.[1]

Characteristics unrelated to need

The examples just used to challenge the fairness of the cost-effectiveness characteristic introduced into the discussion characteristics of the patients concerned that were not directly to do with their need for treatment, or at least not to do with the illness for which the rationing decision had to be made. These included patients' socio-economic circumstances (poor or rich), their age and their degree of disability. This raises a broader question: should characteristics of patients that are not related to their immediate need for treatment affect the rationing decision, and if so in what way?

One point should be disposed of immediately. Some of these characteristics will directly affect treatment effectiveness. For instance, smoking may well impede recovery from certain procedures; hence, on cost-effectiveness grounds alone, it may be sensible to give a lower priority to smokers. But that is not the kind of argument being discussed here. Rather it is to ask whether there might be reasons for discriminating between two patients – for giving one priority over another – even if the effectiveness of a given procedure were the same for both of them. Or it is to ask, if use of the cost-effectiveness characteristic (or indeed any need-related characteristics) has as an unintended consequence discrimination against patients with certain non-need characteristics (such as elderly people, disabled people – or smokers), whether that need-related characteristic should be over-ridden.

---

1. It should be noted that this argument does not apply in the case of non-life-threatening diseases. For in these cases, if other things are equal, then the capacity to gain QALYs is the same for disabled and able-bodied people even if their eventual health status is different. So the cost-per-QALY is identical.

It is easy to think of examples in addition to the ones already discussed where it might be tempting to ration according to characteristics unrelated to need. Tiny Tim versus Scrooge. The unrepentant, militant smoker versus the ex-smoker who succeeded in giving up after an immense personal struggle. The Nobel-prize winner versus the serial killer. Those who have been waiting a long time for treatment versus those who have only recently acquired the need. In each case it is not difficult to think of more or less convincing arguments that could be put forward favouring one over the other in the allocation of medical care, quite independently of cost-effectiveness.

Now few would seriously contend that non-need factors on their own ought to be factors in rationing decisions, if by so doing the outcome would be *negative* discrimination: that is, discrimination against already disadvantaged groups. That would undoubtedly be regarded as inequitable – although, as noted above, in the case of socio-economic status at least, it might be more efficient in the sense of maximising health gain.

However, that is not the end of the argument. Is there a case that some of these non-health factors, particularly those which can lead to political, social and economic disadvantage such as race, gender, income, social class and disability, should be used as the basis for *positive* discrimination in rationing? That is, other things being equal, it could be argued that equity required health care for the poor, for ethnic minorities or for women, for instance, to be given priority over health care for the better off, for the white population or for males – on the grounds that this offered the former some compensation for their disadvantaged position in the wider society.

Another example of a patient characteristic unrelated to need that could be defended as a criterion for rationing concerns dependants. It could be claimed that parents with young children should receive treatment before childless people with otherwise the same need for the treatment. Similarly carers for elderly people, workers, or household bread-winners might be given priority. Even more broadly, some might consider people who make a wider contribution to the community (Nobel-prize winners, political leaders) ought to take priority, while those who 'cost' the community (alcoholics, beggars, criminals) ought to fall to the bottom of the list.

A rather different kind of a case could be made for rationing health care according to desert: that is, as to whether patients are 'deserving' or 'undeserving'. In recent years, this issue has arisen particularly with respect to 'self-induced' diseases. If people deliberately take health risks in the full knowledge of those risks, should they not be held responsible for any adverse health consequences that ensue? Are they not in a sense less deserving than those who contract an illness because of factors entirely beyond their control, and hence should they not be given a lower priority for treatment? Cases that raise these kind of issues and that have recently attracted a great deal of attention concern the treatment of smokers for conditions that have been brought on by smoking; other examples include injuries resulting from dangerous sporting activities, such as skiing; self-inflicted injuries due to drunken driving, and so on.

To ration on these grounds could be defended as being consistent with a general notion of fairness. One of the authors has argued elsewhere that the ways in which the terms 'fairness' or 'equity' are conventionally used often embody concerns about the choices open to the individuals involved (Le Grand, 1991). A situation where one individual is in a worse state than another because of factors entirely beyond that individual's control is commonly regarded as unfair or inequitable; however, if the difference in individual states is the consequence of freely made choices, then the situation is likely to be regarded as fair.

On the other hand, application of this procedure to rationing could present severe difficulties in practice. It is difficult to think of cases where an individual's choices have played no part in her contracting an illness, except possibly for diseases that are entirely genetically transmitted. Pneumonia can result from a walk in the rain; heart attacks from running for a bus, and so on. So use of this characteristic for rationing would require the rationer to make sophisticated judgements as to the exact degree to which an individual was responsible for her condition; an impossible task in most clinical situations, or other settings where rationing decisions have to take place.[2]

---

2. For this reason it has been suggested that this characteristic might be more appropriately applied to the finance side, rather than the delivery side of health care (Le Grand, 1991, pp. 118–24).

Assessment

We thus have a bewildering set of possible candidates for discriminating between people in making rationing decisions over health care. To summarise, these include *need-related characteristics*, such as illness or health deficit, effectiveness and cost-effectiveness; and *characteristics unrelated to need*, such as age, gender, race, socio-economic status, time waiting, number of dependants, and desert.

So what to do? Should rationing between people be based solely on need characteristics? If so, on what interpretation of need? Should characteristics unrelated to need be incorporated into the rationing decision? If so, which ones: socio-economic status, dependants, contribution, desert?

In trying to answer this question it is useful to distinguish between several levels at which the decisions that affect rationing outcomes take place. For patients treated under cost-per-case contracts (usually those of GP fund-holders or those subject to extra-contractual referrals) the rationing decision will be made by the purchaser. For patients treated under block contracts, rationing is a consequence of two levels of decisions: decisions by the budget manager of a provider unit to allocate a certain amount of resources to a specialty within that unit, and the decision by clinicians to allocate those resources within the specialty between patients. The budget manager's decision will itself depend on other resource allocation decisions, notably those incorporated in the block contracts of the purchaser(s) with which the provider has to deal. And, of course, for both cost-per-case and block contracts, the decisions of the purchasers themselves will depend on the overall resource allocation decisions of the central government.

So there are multiple actors involved in the rationing decision. What factors should they consider in making their decisions? *In general, we are unsympathetic to the view that patient characteristics unrelated to need should be incorporated into rationing decisions, whoever is making the relevant decisions.* This is partly for reasons of principle and partly for reasons of pragmatism.

The more philosophical reasons are threefold. The first is the fact that, while few would argue against issues of need playing a role in rationing, most of the arguments concerning the desirability of a role for non-need characteristics are, as we have seen, contested in one way or another. Hence, even if it were agreed that non-need factors should play a role, it would be hard to decide which ones were appropriate, and how they should relate to the need-related characteristics.

The second argument relates to positive discrimination. Given its role as a health service, it seems inappropriate to use the NHS as a device for correcting other social ills, such as poverty or discrimination. If a particular social evil is identified as undesirable, then it should be attacked directly, not by diverting other public services from their primary tasks. The NHS should not be an instrument of social compensation.

The third, and perhaps most powerful, argument derives from the nature of the NHS itself. The original aim of the NHS was to relate treatment to need, and only to need. Put another way, the NHS can be viewed as part of a social contract in which every citizen in need of care has an entitlement to it, regardless of socio-economic status, or any other factor irrelevant to that need.[3] Hence the use of non-need factors to determine who should receive treatment, even if undertaken for the most honourable of motives, would violate that contract.

The pragmatic considerations stem from the fact that, in most cases of rationing, it will be clinicians who are the dominant decision-makers, whether as hospital consultants deciding whom to give priority on a waiting-list, or as GP fundholders, or as public health physicians advising a health authority on priority setting in the main contract or on extra-contractual referrals. Now, clinicians are not trained ethicists; nor are they omniscient. They have neither the skills nor always the information to make the kinds of fine discriminatory judgements that would be necessary if patient characteristics unrelated to need were to be systematically involved in rationing. To argue that clinicians should take factors unrelated

---

3. So, for instance, consider the following from the 1944 White Paper that foreshadowed the NHS:

> 'The Government ... want to ensure that in future every man, woman and child can rely on getting all the advice and treatment and care which they may need in matters of personal health; that what they get shall be the best medical and other facilities available; that their getting these shall not depend on whether they can pay for them, <u>or any other factor irrelevant to the real need.</u>' Cmd 6502, A National Health Service (1944), p.1, emphasis added.

to need into account in their rationing decisions is ultimately to argue for arbitrariness and inconsistency.

On the other hand, clinicians *are* trained to make judgements about the extent of illness and of the effectiveness of treatment. Moreover, increasingly, they are acquiring knowledge of the different costs of treatment and therefore gaining expertise in the area of cost-effectiveness. It is these areas where clinicians' skills lie; and, *in situations where they are the active agents in the process of rationing between people*, rationing procedures have to build on those skills. So the requirements of the reality of rationing procedures in practice would suggest that need-related factors have to be the principal criteria – indeed, except perhaps in special circumstances to be discussed shortly, the only criteria – for making rationing decisions.

One possible qualification to all this concerns the possibility of a tie. If two individuals are determined as equally in need of treatment, but there is not enough for both, then there may be room for some other patient characteristic (such as the existence or otherwise of dependants) to be taken into account. However, even here in many cases the problems over lack of relevant information and/or of the ethical skills necessary to evaluate potentially competing criteria will remain; and it may be that the fairest way to proceed in such a situation would be allocate by a random procedure, such as first come, first served, or, if that were regarded as insufficiently random, by a lottery.

So clinicians commonly have to play a dominant role in rationing between people; and, clinicians' area of specialism concerns illness and effectiveness. These facts, coupled with the more principled arguments outlined above, suggest that need has to be the dominant criterion for rationing between people.

Even if the arguments concerning the primacy of need are accepted, one difficulty remains. Should 'need' be interpreted in terms of the extent of illness, in terms of effectiveness, or in terms of cost-effectiveness of treatment? We have seen that these interpretations may lead to conflicting outcomes in practice: in such situations, which should dominate? Pragmatic considerations offer us little by way of a guide with respect to the difference between the extent of illness and effectiveness, since clinicians should be expert in both; but they might tend to weigh against *cost*-effectiveness. Many clinicians, while prepared to accept that evidence concerning effectiveness should affect their rationing decisions, may be reluctant to do the same with evidence concerning cost-effectiveness, regarding cost considerations as both morally suspect and someone else's business.

Arguments of principle also offer us little guidance with respect to choosing between the extent of illness and effectiveness. However, they do help with respect to effectiveness vs. cost-effectiveness. For the reasons that lead to a concern with effectiveness automatically lead to a concern with cost-effectiveness. Rationing that does not discriminate on the basis of effectiveness is unsatisfactory because it involves a waste of resources: that is, it leads to other needs being unmet. Cost is simply a way of quantifying those unmet needs; so a cost comparison between two procedures states that the application of one of them leads to more (equal or less) unmet need elsewhere than the other. Hence, although the ways in which actual costing procedures may be carried out in practice may be questionable, given that effectiveness is an acceptable criterion for rationing in the first place, there can be no objection in principle to taking cost (measured in some way) into account.

Of course, none of this implies that clinicians are perfect rationers, even in terms of illness, effectiveness or cost-effectiveness. In many cases their knowledge base is sadly out of date, especially when the latest evidence concerning the effectiveness of different kinds of procedures is concerned. Like everyone else, they have their whims and prejudices that distort their judgements; for instance, consultants may be tempted to favour cases that are medically 'interesting' over ones that are more cost-effective but more routine.

However, these difficulties are not insurmountable. If it is felt that clinicians are not up-to-date with respect to the latest evidence concerning effectiveness, then the solution is to provide them with the latest information. To avoid whims, accountability for decision-making can be improved. Finally, if they do not have the right incentives to take cost-effective decisions, then the answer is to change the incentive structure so that they do. GP fundholding is one example of this final strategy; consultants holding the budget for clinical directorates is another.

Conclusion

The argument of this chapter may be summarised as follows. Rationing between people has often to be left to clinicians. Both because of this and because of the fundamental principles that underlay the formation of the NHS, the principles that guide rationing decisions should be based on clinicians' skill and knowledge base: that relating to clinical need. Need may be interpreted either in terms of health deficit or effectiveness; and we believe that there is no general rule that automatically favours one interpretation over another in every case. However, in those cases where effectiveness is the appropriate criterion, it has to be interpreted in terms of cost-effectiveness.

Of course, in practice it may be difficult to prevent clinicians making rationing decisions on the basis of criteria other than need. To do so, appropriate monitoring and accountability procedures will need to be set up. It is perhaps here – in improving the ability of the system effectively to police rationing decisions – that the next stage of the rationing debate should take place.

Chapter 6

Conclusion

The rationing debate tends to polarise those who take part in it. This polarisation occurs, for example, between those who disagree on philosophical grounds as to the appropriate criteria for choosing between people. It also occurs on more practical matters, such as whether it is feasible to develop measures of health gain such as the QALY. But it also polarises opinion on whether *any* strategy for addressing the problem is possible or desirable. Those who believe that progress must be made in making rationing more explicit, systematic and democratic – in our terms, more 'rational' – are probably in the majority, but nevertheless a smaller group of critics argue that such policies are naïve and fundamentally misunderstand the very nature of the NHS.

We believe that there are strong arguments in support of both these positions. It would be hard to advocate a wholesale return to the rationing of resources entirely hidden from public view, with little or no objective intellectual rigour and almost total disregard for the views of the general public. But there is a very real danger that moving too fast in abandoning a system which has sustained the NHS for nearly fifty years could prove equally damaging. The NHS is about more than simply producing health; it acts as a mechanism, and a symbol, of reassurance and social stability. How it achieves this is extremely subtle and quite possibly beyond the ability of any individual to explain satisfactorily.

Another aspect of the delivery of health care militates against 'systematic' policies, whatever their motivation: the highly heterogeneous and contingent nature of medical interventions. Any policy seeking to codify actions based on effectiveness, for instance, will tend to founder on the fact that individuals can very often benefit from procedures which, on average, appear ineffective. This problem has frustrated the attempts of some countries to institute national policies on a 'package' of core services available to all, and where the policy has succeeded (in Oregon), it has been in special circumstances and has remained extremely controversial nevertheless. Furthermore, acknowledging this phenomenon means acknowledging that clinicians are inevitably going to be the final arbiters of individual rationing decisions, leaving national policies which seek to develop appropriate criteria for rationing at this 'micro' level struggling to achieve anything of substance.

Can realistic and workable policies for improving the rationing of health care be devised under these circumstances? We may have no choice. The intense media analysis of all matters concerning the NHS and a steadily more knowledgeable and better informed citizenry have meant that the old implicit system is already vanishing in one important respect: fewer people believe that the NHS can do all that is medically possible for everyone in need. And the reluctance of governments to raise taxes means that significant increases in spending are not an option either.

What is required is to design policies which address the continuing inconsistency and arbitrariness in the rationing of health care, while allaying the growing fears that the NHS is no longer sustainable. In this book we offer two suggestions.

- First, there is a case for specifying at the national level the range of services which, in principle, the NHS is in the business of providing. But, in order to address the issue of heterogeneity, the range of services would be established not on the quantification of the effects on individuals, but on the characteristics of the service which make health care 'special' – fundamental importance, information imbalance and unpredictability. This range of services would not be a 'core package', but rather *all* those services which are relevant to a health care system. The goal would be to reintroduce a sense of geographical equity and reassurance into the NHS: no health authority would be allowed to avoid provision of at least some level of service; the actual level of provision, highly contingent on local circumstances, would be left to local discretion.
- Second, such a range of services would almost certainly be capable of providing more benefit to individuals than a publicly financed system could afford. In these circumstances, there will remain a need to establish a fair means of distributing these benefits between the rival claims on them – in other words, fair criteria will need to be established for

rationing resources. For reasons of principle and pragmatism, we support need-related criteria – extent of ill health and cost-effectiveness – as appropriate for rationing health care. In principle, they are closer to the avowed function of the NHS; with respect to pragmatism, we argue that clinicians are inevitably going to be the ultimate rationers and therefore should only discriminate on the basis of their expertise. How these criteria are weighted should be left up to the individual clinician and the individual case. What we do need is improved systems of monitoring so that the decisions of the medical profession can be held to account more successfully in the future.

These proposals are made in the spirit of improving a system which in many ways has worked remarkably well. Attempts to be more systematic, explicit and democratic may not always result in anticipated improvements; reforms to the system of rationing in the NHS should be made with caution and with due regard for the limits of knowledge.

References

H. Aaron and W. Schwartz (1984), *The Painful Prescription: Rationing hospital care*, The Brookings Institution, Washington DC.

K. Arrow (1963), 'Uncertainty and the welfare economics of medical care', *American Economic Review*, 53, pp. 941–73.

Audit Commission (1995), *Briefing on GP Fundholding*, London.

V. Beardshaw and R. Robinson (1990), *New for Old? Prospects for nursing in the 1990s*, Research Report No. 8, King's Fund Institute, London.

J. Bell and S. Mendus (1988), *Philosophy and Medical Welfare*, Cambridge University Press, Cambridge.

G. Bevan and B. Devlin (1994), *All Free Health Care Must Be Effective: Limiting medical practice variation*, Social Market Foundation Memorandum No. 4, February.

S. Bjork and P. Rosen (1993), Setting health care priorities in Sweden: the politician's point of view', *Health Policy*, 26, pp. 141–4.

A. Bowling (1993), *What People Say about Prioritising Health Services*, King's Fund Centre, London.

D. Brindle (1994), 'Call to clarify rights to NHS treatment', *The Guardian*, 28 April, p. 9.

British Medical Association (1994), *Equal access to NHS treatment*, BMA press statement, 13 January 1994.

BMJ (1993), *Rationing in Action*, BMJ Publishing Group, London.

D. Callahan (1994), *What Kind of Life?*, Georgetown University Press, Washington DC.

L. Churchill (1987), *Rationing Health Care in America: Perceptions and principles of justice*, University of Notre Dame Press, Notre Dame, Indiana.

Cmd 6502 (1944), *A National Health Service*, HMSO, London.

Cmd 9663 (1956), *Report of the Committee of Inquiry into the Cost of the National Health Service*, HMSO, London.

M. Cooper (1995), 'Core services and the New Zealand health reforms', in R. Maxwell (ed.) *Rationing Health Care*, Churchill Livingstone, London (Special edition of the *British Medical Bulletin*, 51(4), pp. 799–807).

M. Crail (1995), 'Rational judgements', *Health Service Journal*, 7 September, p. 12.

J. Cullis and P. West (1979), *The Economics of Health: An introduction*, Martin Robertson.

A. Culyer (1971), 'The nature of the commodity "health care" and its efficient allocation', *Oxford Economic Papers*, 23, pp. 189–211.

A. Culyer (1988), 'Inequality of health services is, in general, desirable', in D. Green (ed.) *Acceptable Inequalities*, Institute of Economic Affairs, London.

A. Culyer (1995), 'Need: the idea won't do – but we still need it', *Social Science and Medicine* 40(6), pp. 727–30.

A. Culyer and A. Wagstaff (1992), *Need, Equity and Equality in Health and Health Care*, Discussion Paper 95, Centre for Health Economics, University of York.

A. Culyer and A. Wagstaff (1993), 'Equity and equality in health and health care', *Journal of Health Economics*, 12, pp. 431–57.

N. Daniels (1985), *Just Health Care*, Cambridge University Press, Cambridge.
M. Dean (1991), 'The Oregon trail reaches Britain', *The Lancet*, 338, pp. 1133–4.
M. Dean (1994), 'Rationing care by age deemed unfair', *The Lancet*, 343, p. 1278.
Department of Health (1993a), *Additions to the list of items which may not be supplied on NHS prescription*, Press Release H93/989, 11 October.
Department of Health (1993b), *Smokers denied treatment*, Press Release H93/990, 11 October.
Department of Health (1993c), *Self-medication encourages individual commitment to health*, Press Release H93/1092, 29 November.
Department of Health (1994), *Virginia Bottomley spells out policy on NHS treatment for elderly people*, Press Release 94/182, 15 April.
Department of Health (1995), *Developing and Implementing Eligibility Criteria for Continuing Care: A checklist for purchasers*, DoH, London.
C. Donaldson (1993), 'Economics of priority setting: let's ration rationally!', in *Rationing in Action*, BMJ Publishing Group, London.
L. Doyal and I. Gough (1991), *A Theory of Human Need*, Macmillan, London.
N. Dudley and E. Burns (1990), 'The influence of age on policies for admission and thrombolysis in Coronary Care Units in the UK', *Age and Aging*, 21, pp. 95–8.
P. Dunleavy and B. O'Leary (1978), *Theories of the State: The politics of liberal democray*, MacMillan Education, London.
A. Dunning (1992), *Report of the Government Committee on Choices in Health Care*, Ministry of Welfare, Health and Cultural Affairs, Rijswijk, The Netherlands.
R. Dworkin (1994), 'Will Clinton's plan be fair?', *New York Review*, 13 January, pp. 20–5.
H. Feger (1993), 'Practice where patients advise on care rationing', *Pulse*, 53 (3 April), p. 22.
D. Fox and H. Leichter (1991), 'Rationing care in Oregon: the new accountability', *Health Affairs*, 10 (Summer), pp. 7–27.
S. Frankel and R. West (1993) (eds.), *Rationing and Rationality in the National Health Service: The persistence of waiting lists*, Macmillan, London.
B. Fuchs and M. Merlis (1993), *Health Care Reform: President Clinton's Health Security Act*, Congressional Research Service, The Library of Congress, Washington.
S. Giles (1993), 'Rationing scheme will exclude minor illnesses from NHS', *Health Service Journal*, 26 August, p. 7.
J. Grimshaw and A. Hutchinson (1995), 'Clinical Practice Guidelines – do they enhance value for money in health care?', in R. Maxwell (ed.) *Rationing Health Care*, Churchill Livingstone, London (Special edition of the *British Medical Bulletin*, 51(4), pp. 927–40).
C. Ham (1985), *Health Policy in Britain*, 2nd edition, Macmillan, London.
C. Ham (1993), 'Priority setting in the NHS: reports from six districts', *BMJ*, 307, pp. 435–8.
J. Harris (1988), 'More and better justice', in Bell and Mendus (1988), *Philosophy and Medical Welfare*, Cambridge University Press, Cambridge.
A. Harrison (ed.) (1992), *Health Care UK 1991*, King's Fund Institute, London.
A. Harrison (ed.) (1993), *Health Care UK 1992/93*, King's Fund Institute, London.
A. Harrison (ed.) (1994), *Health Care UK 1993/94*, King's Fund Institute, London.
S. Harrison (1988), *Managing the NHS: Shifting the frontier?*, Chapman and Hall, London.

S. Harrison and D. Hunter (1994), *Rationing Health Care*, Institute for Public Policy Research, London.

Health Care and Medical Priorities Commission (1993), *No Easy Choices – The difficult priorities of health care*, Ministry of Health and Social Affairs, Stockholm.

Healthcare 2000 (1995), *UK Health and Healthcare Services: Challenges and policy options*, Healthcare 2000, London.

C. Heginbotham (1993), 'Health care priority setting: a survey of doctors, managers and the general public', in BMJ (1993), *Rationing in Action*, BMJ Publishing Group, London.

T. Hickish, I. Smith, S. Ashley and G. Middleton (1995) 'Chemotherapy for elderly patients with lung cancer', *The Lancet*, 346, August 26.

F. Honigsbaum, J. Calltorp, C. Ham and S. Holmström (1995), *Priority Setting Processes for Healthcare*, Radcliffe Medical Press, Oxford.

House of Commons Health Committee, First Report (1995), *Priority Setting in the NHS: Purchasing*, Session 1994–95, 134–1, HMSO, London.

D. Hunter (1991), 'Pain of going public', *Health Service Journal*, 101 (29 August), p. 20.

D. Hunter (1993), *Rationing Dilemmas in Health Care*, Research Paper 8, NAHAT, Birmingham.

D. Hunter (1994), 'Are we being effective?', *Health Service Journal*, 16 June, p. 23.

D. Hunter and C. Webster (1992), 'Here we go again', *Health Service Journal*, 5 March, pp. 26–7.

R. Jarvis (1994), 'Health care planning: an ethical dimension?', *Bulletin of Medical Ethics*, February, pp. 17–18.

C. Jones (1950), *Cabinet Committee on the National Health Service: Enquiry into the Financial Workings of the Service – Report by Sir Cyril Jones*. CAB 134/518, Public Records Office, London.

K. Judge and N. Mays (1994), 'Allocating resources for health and social care in England', *BMJ*, 308, pp. 1363–6.

J. Kitzhaber and A.M. Kenny (1995), 'On the Oregon trail', in R. Maxwell (ed.) *Rationing Health Care*, Churchill Livingstone, London (Special edition of the *British Medical Bulletin*, 51(4), pp. 808–18).

H. Klarman, J. Francis and G. Rosenthal (1968), 'Cost-effectiveness applied to the treatment of chronic renal disease', *Medical Care*, 6, 48–54.

R. Klein (1991), 'On the Oregon trail: rationing health care', *BMJ*, 302, pp. 1–2.

R. Klein (1993a), 'Dimensions of rationing: who should do what?', *BMJ*, 307, pp. 309–11.

R. Klein (1993b), 'The NHS: church or garage?', in A. Harrison (ed.) *Health Care UK 1992/93*, King's Fund Institute, London.

R. Klein (1994), 'Can we restrict the health care menu?', *Health Policy*, 27, pp. 103–12.

R. Klein (1995), *The New Politics of the NHS*, 3rd edn., Longman, London.

R. Klein and S. Redmayne (1992), *Patterns of Priorities: A study of the purchasing and rationing policies of health authorities*, NAHAT Research Paper 7, NAHAT, Birmingham.

J. Le Grand (1991), *Equity and Choice: An essay in economics and applied philosophy*, HarperCollins (now Routledge), London.

P. Lewis and M. Charney (1989), 'Which of two individuals do you treat when only their ages are different and you cannot treat both?', *Journal of Medical Ethics*, 15, pp. 28–32.

C. Lindblom (1979), 'Still muddling, not yet through', *Public Administration Review*, 39 (November/December), pp. 517–26.
J. Lubitz and G. Riley (1993), 'Trends in Medicare payments in the last year of life', *New England Journal of Medicine*, 328, pp. 1092–6.
A. McGuire, J. Henderson and G. Mooney (1988) *The Economics of Health Care: An introductory text*, Routledge & Kegan Paul, London.
G. Majone (1989), *Evidence, Argument and Persuasion in the Policy Process*, Yale University Press, New Haven.
R. Maxwell (ed.) (1995), *Rationing Health Care*, Churchill Livingstone, London. (Special edition of the *British Medical Bulletin*, 51(4)).
D. Mechanic (1992), 'Professional judgement and the rationing of medical care' *University of Pennsylvania Law Review*, 140, pp. 1713–54.
D. Mechanic (1995), 'Dilemmas in rationing health care services: the case for implicit rationing', *BMJ*, 310, pp. 1655–9.
G. Mooney (1986) *Economics, Medicine and Health Care*, Wheatsheaf, Brighton.
G. Mooney (1994), 'What else do we want from our health services?', *Social Science and Medicine*, 39, pp. 151–4.
P. Mullen (1995), *Is Health Care Rationing Really Necessary?*, Discussion Paper 36, Health Services Management Centre, University of Birmingham, Birmingham.
National Advisory Committee on Core Health and Disability Services (1994), *Core Services 1993/4, First Report*, Government Printing Office, New Zealand.
National Confidential Enquiry into Perioperative Deaths (1993), *Report 1991/2*, NCEPOD, London.
B. New (1993), 'Accountability and control in the NHS', in A. Harrison (ed.) *Health Care UK 1992/93*, King's Fund Institute, London.
NHS Management Executive (1992), *Local Voices: The views of local people in purchasing for health*, London.
J.E. Powell (1966), *Medicine and Politics*, Pitman Medical Publishing, London.
J. Rawls (1972), *A Theory of Justice*, Oxford University Press, Oxford.
S. Redmayne (1995), *Reshaping the NHS: Strategies, priorities and resource allocation*, NAHAT Research Paper 16, NAHAT, Birmingham.
S. Redmayne and R. Klein (1993), 'Rationing in practice: the case of *in vitro* fertilisation', *BMJ*, 306, pp. 1521–4.
S. Redmayne, R. Klein and P. Day (1993), *Sharing Out Resources: Purchasing and priority setting in the NHS*, NAHAT Research Paper 11, NAHAT, Birmingham.
R. Rhodes (1992), *Health Care Politics, Policy and Distributive Justice: The ironic triumph*, State University of New York Press, New York.
R. Robinson (1993), 'Purchasing, priorities and rationing', in A. Harrison (ed.) *Health Care UK 1992/93*, King's Fund Institute, London.
R. Robinson and B. New (1992), 'Health economics and economists in the NHS', *BMJ*, 305, p. 1361.
A. Shaw (1994), 'In defence of ageism', *Journal of Medical Ethics*, 20, pp. 188–91.
T. Sheldon and A. Maynard (1993), 'Is rationing inevitable?', in BMJ (1993), *Rationing in Action*, BMJ Publishing Group, London.

R. Smith (1991), 'Where is the wisdom...? The poverty of medical evidence', *BMJ*, 303, pp. 798–9.

M. Strosberg, J. Wiener, R. Baker and I. Fein (eds.) (1992), *Rationing America's Medical Care: The Oregon plan and beyond*, The Brooking's Institution, Washington DC.

L. Turnberg (1994), *Ensuring Equity and Quality of Care for Elderly People*, The Royal College of Physicians of London, London.

L. Turnberg (1995), *Setting Priorities in the NHS: A framework for decision-making*, The Royal College of Physicians of London, London.

M. Underwood, J. Bailey, M. Shiu, R. Higgs and J. Garfield (1993), 'Should smokers be offered coronary bypass surgery?', *BMJ*, 306, pp. 1047–50.

W. van de Ven (1995), 'Choices in health care: a contribution from the Netherlands', in R. Maxwell (ed.) *Rationing Health Care*, Churchill Livingstone, London (Special edition of the *British Medical Bulletin*, 51(4), pp. 781–90).

M. Whitehead (1994), 'Who cares about equity in the NHS?', *BMJ*, 308, pp. 1284–7.

A. Williams (1978), '"Need" – an economic exegesis', reprinted in A. Culyer (ed.) (1991), *The Economics of Health*, Vol.1, Edward Elgar, Aldershot.

A. Williams (1985), 'Economics of coronary artery by-pass grafting' *BMJ*, 291, pp. 326–9.

A. Williams (1988), 'Ethics and efficiency in the provision of health care', in Bell and Mendus (eds.) *Philosophy and Medical Welfare*, Cambridge University Press, Cambridge.

A. Williams (1989), *Creating a Health Care Market: Ideology, efficiency, ethics and clinical freedom*, NHS White Paper Occasional Paper 5, Centre for Health Economics, University of York.

Working Group to the Director of Research and Development of the NHS Management Executive (1993), 'What do we mean by appropriate health care?', *Quality in Health Care*, 2, pp. 117–23.